Fariza Halimova

Reproductive health of women of different ethnic groups

Fariza Halimova

Reproductive health of women of different ethnic groups

ScienciaScripts

Imprint
Any brand names and product names mentioned in this book are subject to trademark, brand or patent protection and are trademarks or registered trademarks of their respective holders. The use of brand names, product names, common names, trade names, product descriptions etc. even without a particular marking in this work is in no way to be construed to mean that such names may be regarded as unrestricted in respect of trademark and brand protection legislation and could thus be used by anyone.

Cover image: www.ingimage.com

This book is a translation from the original published under ISBN 978-620-4-98023-2.

Publisher:
Sciencia Scripts
is a trademark of
Dodo Books Indian Ocean Ltd. and OmniScriptum S.R.L publishing group

120 High Road, East Finchley, London, N2 9ED, United Kingdom
Str. Armeneasca 28/1, office 1, Chisinau MD-2012, Republic of Moldova, Europe
Printed at: see last page
ISBN: 978-620-7-62337-2

FARIZA TURSUNBAEVNA KHALIMOVA

REPRODUCTIVE HEALTH OF WOMEN OF DIFFERENT ETHNIC GROUPS

TABLE OF CONTENTS

Reproductive health stands out from the general health problem because of its social and political significance. At the same time, the analysis of domestic and foreign literature shows that the protection of women's reproductive health is one of the most important medical and social problems of state importance, since women's reproductive health is the main potential for reproduction of the country's population, its demographic resource, without which neither economic nor social growth of the state is possible [30; 5; 182]. Both physiological indicators of reproductive health and the nature of its disorders depend on the climatic, geographical and environmental conditions in which a woman lives, on her ethnicity [3; 226; 141].

The socio-economic and political changes that have been taking place in Russia over the past 25 years have also affected demographic processes and have had an impact on reproductive, sexual and migratory behaviour of people, on family and marriage relations - [5], and many of the problems and trends related to fertility and reproductive health of the population are becoming relevant not only in Russia, but also in many other CIS countries, including the Republic of Tajikistan - [46; 14].

The last decades of the past century have been characterised by significant advances in the diagnosis and treatment of various forms of fertility disorders [3; 215]. At the same time, of particular importance is the currently established connection between disorders of reproductive function of the female organism and its racial and ethnic characteristics, climatic-geographical, socio-economic and environmental conditions in which a woman lives -[145; 226].

As shown by numerous studies, in the process of evolution under the influence of natural selection, as well as under the influence of various environmental conditions, the representatives of different ethnic groups formed and hereditarily fixed structural and functional features inherent only to them, which had an adaptive value, determined the anthropological type and influenced the reproductive function [162; 215; 216; 160; 186].

Traditionally and quite justifiably, the structure of reproductive disorders is characterised by anatomical causes, infectious agents, endocrine factors, genetic and immunological causes. However, despite the progress achieved well , the problems of pregnancy preservation are still far from being definitively solved [26; 172]. The importance of hormonal status in the formation of reproductive health is being intensively studied, and population features of hormonal support of reproductive functions remain one of the topical areas of research.

The possibility of adequate adaptation of a woman's organism to the environment is largely provided by the influence of sex hormones, the change in the concentration of which leads to a significant difference in the humoral regulation of body functions [26; 34; 194; 212]. At the same time, reproductive disorders in women (infertility, pregnancy failure, stillbirth, etc.) are most often associated with endocrine pathology. For example, endocrine female infertility accounts for about 30-40% in the structure of infertile marriage [32].

Human population genetics opens new promising directions for the assessment of population health before modern medical science. At present, the relationship between population genetic and demographic characteristics of populations that determine their gene pools and various types of reproductive pathology has been proved - [40]. However, the number of these studies is still small. The influence of genetic characteristics on women's reproductive health has not yet been adequately covered in the scientific literature, and the available data are often contradictory - [50]. The study of the role of immunogenetic factors in reproductive disorders is considered promising from the point of view of predicting reproductive disorders and combating infertility, but this aspect of the study of the problem is still far from the final disclosure of the role of immunogenetics in the formation of reproductive health. Reproductive immunology, on the one hand, requires an in-depth deciphering of immunological mechanisms and, on the other hand, needs reliable markers of immunopathological conditions associated with reproductive disorders. The frequency of the combination of autoimmune pathology and reproductive disorders needs to be assessed from a population perspective. The example of antiphospholipid reaction shows the prospect of developing scales for quantitative risk assessment of reproductive disorders, which would make it possible to start creating and widely implementing a system of effective measures for their prevention.

The issues of immunogenetics based on HLA-genotyping are considered to be particularly relevant, which already today bring results that are actively implemented in clinical practice - [140; 139].

Based on the successes of immunogenetics, as well as in connection with the rapid development of immunity science in general, the study of immunology of the reproductive process occurring in the female body has advanced significantly in recent years and is recognised as one of the most promising directions in solving the problems of reproductive disorders [27; 189]. The development of modern knowledge of immune system cells and molecular mechanisms of their interaction, supplemented by the growth of diagnostic technologies, allows us to penetrate deeper into the essence of immunological shifts accompanying reproduction and to work successfully towards the development of effective therapeutic measures related to this area of reproductive disorders [37; 156; 221].

Studies on the autoimmune processes accompanying the realisation of reproductive functions are developing, as it has been established that about but 20% of women with habitual pregnancy failure and pregnancy complications have autoimmune disorders caused by antiphospholipid antibodies, have high rates of antinuclear antibodies, as well as antibodies to thyroid components [31; 127; 179].

All these problems, despite their active development, still have a lot of white spots, while the issues related to the development of risk criteria for violations of women's reproductive health and allowing to predict their development at the prenosological level remain the most urgent.

Purpose of the study: to test the cluster-population approach to assessing the risk of reproductive health disorders in women of fertile age in the Russian and Tajik populations and to develop quantitative criteria for such assessment at the prenosological stage.

In order to achieve the stated objective, the following were formulated

research objectives:

1. To clarify physiological norms and identify population features in women of fertile age in the Russian and Tajik populations, taking into account immunogenetic traits, hormonal and immune status data.

2. On the basis of informative immunogenetic, hormonal and immunological traits, to conduct a cluster analysis of populations of Russian and Tajik women to identify features associated with favourable and unfavourable obstetric history.
3. to characterise the hormonal status of women in the Russian and Tajik populations at risk of reproductive disorders in order to identify quantitative shifts in hormones associated with the reproductive process.
4. to characterise the immune status of women of Russian and Tajik populations at risk of reproductive disorders in order to identify quantitative shifts in immune system cells and immuno glo bulins of different classes associated with the reproductive process.
5. To characterise the autoimmune component in women of Russian and Tajik populations at risk of reproductive disorders in order to identify quantitative shifts in autoantibodies potentially affecting the reproductive process.
6. To create a system of integral risk assessment of reproductive health disorders in women of the Russian and Tajik populations, to develop algorithms for its use, and to test this system on a cohort of unborn women with subsequent follow-up in catamnesis.

Scientific novelty of the study

For the first time, methodological approaches to assessing the risk of reproductive health disorders in women of childbearing age in the Russian and Tajik populations and quantitative criteria for such assessment at the prenosological stage were presented on a reliably large clinical material.

In the process of performing the research for the first time:

- specified physiological norms for the content of hormones, indicators of immune status and autoimmune process in the blood, taking into account the belonging of women to the Russian or Tajik populations;

- The high efficiency of the population cluster approach in analysing women's reproductive health disorders and identifying risk markers for such disorders has been shown;

- It has been established that populations of Russian and Tajik women are characterised by different risk markers for reproductive disorders. ;

- It has been confirmed that a set of allelic variants unfavourable for reproductive health, in particular, HLA-DRB1*04 and HLA-DQA1*0103 genes, is associated with reproductive disorders regardless of a woman's population affiliation ;

- It is shown that in the population of Russian women with reproductive disorders, two risk groups can be distinguished, one of which is dominated by immunological changes, including autoimmune changes, and the other has hormonal shifts;

- It is also shown that in the population of Tajik women with impaired reproductive function in one of the risk groups a combination of immunological shifts, different in nature from those in Russian women, prevails, while in the other risk group autoimmune shifts characteristic of antiphospholipid reactions are observed;

- criterion ranges of deviations of each informative indicator in each population of women with reproductive disorders were determined;

- integral markers of reproductive disorders have been developed for each of the 4 risk groups, ranges of prognostically significant values of these markers have been established, and their prognostic efficiency has been proved.

CHAPTER 1. CURRENT STATE OF THE PROBLEM OF ASSESSING REPRODUCTIVE HEALTH DISORDERS IN WOMEN OF FERTILE AGE

1.1 Concept and criteria for evaluating reproductive labour women's health

According to the WHO definition: "Reproductive health is a state of complete physical, mental and social well-being and not merely the absence of disease or infirmity in all areas relating to the reproductive system, its functions and processes, including reproduction and harmony in psychosocial relationships within the family. Population health, including reproductive health, is determined by the economic and social situation of the population, demographic processes, and environmental living conditions - [62].

In the early 1990s Russia entered a period of prolonged depopulation, one of the main reasons for which was the ultra-low birth rate - [7]. In general, in 1995 - 2008, the population loss in Russia totalled 5.7 million people, and since 2009 there has been an increase, which in 2014 amounted to 0.9 million people. One ko, the experts of the National Research University Higher School of Economics in the future predict the instability of the trend of natural increase, and the prospects for changes in the number of the population of Russia will be largely associated with migration processes - [76].

In this connection, the concept of demographic policy of the Russian Federation for the period up to 2025, approved by Presidential Decree No. 1351 of 9 October 2007, identified the strengthening of reproductive health and the institution of the family as priority areas of

State policy, since not only the level of fertility but also the viability of future generations depends on them - [56].

A woman's reproductive health implies the absence of reproductive system diseases, the ability to reproduce offspring and determines the number of children in a family: today 65.5 per cent of families among Russians have one child and only 12.9 per cent have three or more children. Among the total population of Russia, the number of women is more than 53 per cent, of which 27.5 per cent (36 million) are of reproductive age. However, according to projections, the number of women in the most active reproductive age (20-29 years old) may drop to 7.5 million by 2021, down from 11 million in 2014. There is also a deformation of the age structure of women of fertile age: an increase in the average age of both all women giving birth (up to 27.1 years) and first-born women (up to 24.7 years) and a shift in the peak of fertility from the 20-24 age group to the 25-29 age group [7].

Trends in fertility factors in the Russian Federation correspond to global trends, but have their own specifics. First of all, it is the devaluation of the insti tute of the family, as evidenced by a 15 per cent decline in marriage rates (from 10.6 per cent in 1980 to 9.2 per cent in 2011) and a high divorce rate (4.7 per cent in 2011). In modern Russia, every second marriage breaks up and every third child is born to an unmarried woman. The transformation of reproductive behaviour, which is characterised by the spread of early sexual debut, loyalty to changing partners, use of low-efficiency contraception and a decline in childbearing attitudes to the point of conscious refusal to give birth - "child free" - is a consequence of the sexual revolution taking place in Russia since the late 1980s, as described by Pitirim Sorokin in 1954 for

American society. As a consequence, only 5% of families in modern Russia have three or more children - [52].

Assessment of the components of reproductive health and reproductive behaviour is inextricably linked to population reproduction. To maintain the population at least at the existing level, a fertility rate of 2.15 is required. Today it is only 1.17 in Russia. Analysing the level of birth rate, abortions, morbidity, it is easy to conclude that almost every region of Russia needs not just stabilisation and population growth, but the creation of conditions for improving the demographic situation [66].

Many of the outlined problems and trends related to fertility and reproductive health of the population are registered not only in Russia, but also in many other CIS countries.

Thus, demographic problems and reproductive health issues are becoming increasingly acute year after year in the Central Asian region and, especially, in the Republic of Tajikistan [8]. After gaining independence in 1999, the Republic of Tajikistan faced major problems inherent in the transition period, which were further exacerbated by political instability and civil war (1992). Tajikistan was the poorest country among all other republics of the former Soviet Union before it gained its independence. During the years of independence, despite significant difficulties in its socio-economic status, the country, with the support of the international community, has taken serious measures to develop comprehensive action to protect women's health; it has ratified important international documents on the protection of women's and children's rights; it has developed a legislative framework for maternal and child health care; and it has established a reproductive health-care service. In 2002, the Government adopted the Reproductive Health and Reproductive Rights Act. . The problems of public health protection are reflected in strategic documents "Strategy of the Republic of Tajikistan on the protection of public health for the period up to 2010" and others. - [56].

The decline in the birth rate in various countries leads to a reduction in the population and, consequently, to a decrease in the share of young people in its structure, which is a significant demographic risk to a country's development. It is manifested, first and foremost, in a decline in the creative potential of young people. The need to ensure demographic security pass , the transition to innovative development determines the relevance of research into the reproductive behaviour of the population and the factors that determine it [52, 86].

Women's reproductive health depends on many factors: heredity, lifestyle, occupational hazards, and diseases of various organs and systems. In Russia, Tajikistan and other CIS countries, women's reproductive health is deteriorating: the absolute number of healthy women does not exceed 6 per cent. The reproductive situation is aggravated by the increasing incidence of gynaecological diseases, including sexually transmitted infections, a consistently high rate of abortions, and infertility [7, 63].

An important social factor that can have a profound impact on reproductive health is socioeconomic status. A number of socio-economic factors, such as a woman's educational status, per capita income, job availability, age at first marriage, life expectancy and infant mortality, have been reported by sociologists as indicators associated with fertility - [126]. Low socioeconomic status with aggravating circumstances, sources of stress such as malnutrition and financial hardship have been found to affect a woman's ovarian reserve, which should be kept in mind in the approach to infertile patients - [126].

A social factor such as a woman's employment status before or during pregnancy plays an important role and has been associated with a range of other factors, including the woman's age, pre-pregnancy body mass index men , pregnancy intentions, smoking, alcohol consumption, and income received. Employment status was significantly associated with many common risk factors for adverse pregnancy outcomes - [178].

Given this variety of factors influencing a woman's reproductive health, a number of authors conclude that there is a need for interdisciplinary approaches to improving maternal and reproductive health and pregnancy outcomes for women who are disadvantaged in terms of education, place of residence, fertility and access to medical cyns com services - [201].

The causes of reproductive disorders are extremely diverse and not always clearly defined. As mentioned above, they include a number of social environmental factors: bad habits, negative factors of the industrial environment, unfulfilled family life, exhausting physical labour, stressful situations, etc. [90]. - [90]. The risk factors of reproductive disorders in modern conditions include increasing maternal age, obesity, smoking, alcohol, existing pathology and anatomical anomalies of the reproductive system [120]. Medical factors are singled out separately: genetic breakdowns of karyotypes of parents, embryo, endocrine system disorders, pathology of uterine development, infectious diseases, previous abortions, stillbirths, etc. [90]. - [90].

In the Russian Federation, 12 million women in the entire female population suffer from infertility, and the incidence of pregnancy failure ranges from 10-25% of all pregnancies [65, 180]. The proportion of infertile marriages is 12-30% and has no tendency to decrease, so it is necessary to further search for ways to diagnose and treat infertility and non-pregnancy - [57]. Authors from the Republic of Kazakhstan indicate a figure of 12% of infertile marriages, commenting that many infertile individuals end up out of wedlock, which makes the true incidence of infertility even higher. At the same time, experts from the World Health Organisation believe that the 15% rate of infertile marriages is a serious public health problem [6].

According to O.I. Apolikhin, N.G. Moskaleva, V.A. Komarova [5], there are two possible ways of solving the problem of improving reproductive health of the nation - extensive and intensive. The extensive way involves treatment of existing diseases and their complications, the so-called tertiary prophylactics, which requires large investments in medical care. This way is costly but necessary, and today it is successfully implemented in federal head centres providing high-tech logical and specialised lised medical care. The main point of the intensive pathway is health preservation, primary prevention, health education work , and active involvement of the individual in taking care of his or her own health. In the context of the creation of new medical technologies, the optimal way is to strengthen disease prevention. Early detection of diseases and the promotion of a healthy lifestyle are highly effective and low-cost measures. Such a model of health care was already created in Russia in 1918 by N.A. Semashko. It was based on unified principles of organisation and centralisation of the health care system; equal accessibility of health care for all citizens; priority attention to childhood and motherhood; unity of prevention and treatment; elimination of social bases of disease ; involvement of the public in health care. Raising awareness and responsible attitude to health is of particular importance nowadays, including through economic incentives (for example, individualisation of insurance). Effective programmes should be considered to be those that, at minimal cost, produce maximum social results measured in the improvement of the quality of life of the country's population and its demographic health indicators [5].

For example, the development of an extensive pathway to improve reproductive ive health in low- and middle-income countries has shown that, in the absence of adequate health care, maternal and newborn illnesses contribute to high mortality rates. Combining demand and service delivery strategies is a major challenge. The implementation of these interventions has had a significant impact on reducing stillbirths, perinatal and neonatal mortality - [208].

At the same time, in order to implement the available reserves, the regions, in addition to the general measures envisaged by State programmes for the protection of reproductive duc health, need to focus their efforts on specific tasks. Each group of territories is characterised by its own problems of reproductive health, leading, on the one hand, to the under-fulfilment of women's reproductive plans due to infertility and, on the other hand, to the loss of desired children due to spontaneous abortions, late abortions and stillbirth [47].

Taking into account the existing knowledge, a certain range of priority directions in solving the problems of preserving reproductive health has been outlined. These are, first of all, the reduction and prevention of maternal and perinatal mortality, the reorientation of women from abortion as the main method of birth control to modern effective means of contraception, sexual education aimed at preventing unwanted pregnancies and the prevention of sexually transmitted diseases - [106].

It should also be taken into account that 40-46% of 100 childless couples do not have children due to male infertility, which is associated with genetics, sexually transmitted infections, the influence of harmful environmental factors, working conditions and bad habits on male reproductive health. The numerical facts convincingly prove the importance of careful attitude to reproductive health of not only women, but also men - [106, 223].

In order to identify regionally specific problems related to the preservation of reproductive functions, special attention should be paid to analysing existing and developing new criteria for assessing reproductive health.

According to modern estimates, the characterisation of a woman's reproductive health as an environmental diagnostic criterion includes at least 10 main indicators:

(1) threatened abortion;

(2) toxicity goats 2nd half of pregnancy;

(3) spontaneous abortions (termination of pregnancy men before 20 weeks);

(4) preterm labour (termination of pregnancy before 37 weeks);

(5) premature expulsion of fetal waters;

(6) anomalies of labour;

(7) perinatal pathology and mortality;

(8) infant mortality;

(9) neonatal pathology;

(10) congenital malformations - [62]. At the same time, maternal and infant mortality should be considered the most important indicator of reproductive health of the population [- 6].

However, according to A.K.Lawson, E.E.Marsh - [183], clinical medical studies aimed at determining the criteria of reproductive health disorders often ignore the individual characteristics of women and, most importantly, their population affiliation.

1.2 Influence of ethnic and climatic-geographical factors on women's reproductive health

The study of adaptation processes of different ethnic groups to climatic and geographical environmental conditions is a priority in the field of biomedical research [2, 17, 45, 51, 189]. Ethnos is defined as "a group of people speaking the same language, recognising their common origin, possessing a set of customs, way of life, kept and sanctified by tradition and distinguishing it from those of other groups" - [33, 38].

Numerous studies show that inhabitants of different geographic fical regions differ from each other in morphofunctional functional characteristics, basic, protein, lipid and mineral metabolism, enzyme and hormonal status, genetic apparatus of the cell, and reproductive functions. These signs are especially pronounced in inhabitants of regions with extreme environmental conditions [21, 30, 41, 68, 93, 139] or in case of global changes [173, 179, 199].

Numerous studies conducted by modern domestic and foreign authors testify that centuries of living va of human populations in habitual habitat conditions determined not only their appearance and cultural features, but also specific morphofunction cyo nal characteristics, peculiarities of vital activity of the organism as a whole. There is reason to believe that most of the most important features of aborigines of different climatogeographic regions were formed at the dawn of human history, i.e. in those epochs when human dependence on the impact of natural habitat was still very high - [61, 102].

Adaptive changes in morpho-physiological structures resulting from mutations useful for life activity in changed conditions were fixed by natural selection while preserving the main genetic traits that characterise humans. With the development of social production, the relationship between man and nature is increasingly mediated by social relations - [50].

In the literature there is information about the existence of ethnic differences of the most important physiological constants of the organism in the functioning not only of individual enzyme systems, but also in the reactions of the neuroimmunoendocrine system to the impact of inadequate exogenous and endogenous factors - [70, 154, 186].

The article by N.A. Aghajanian and I.I. Manakova [1] presents a review of data on morphofunctional features and course of diseases in individuals with different ethnic and racial affiliation. It is shown that these features are caused le by genetic, cultural, socio-economic and environmental factors .

The same, in particular, is discussed in the book by N.G.Gomboeva [29] on the example of analysing the health, demographic situation, adaptation of different ethnic groups (Russians, Buryats) of Eastern Transbaikalia.

The reproductive function of the female organism is particularly sensitive to the effects of harmful environmental factors of any, even small, intensity, including subthreshold ones [4, 64].

From the point of view of survival of a biological species, the reproductive system serves as an instrument of natural selection as a result of which a significant number of non-viable embryos are eliminated - [83, 166].

The results of studies by D.A.Hojamuradova and T.A.Nazarenko [101] confirm not only the heterogeneity and complexity of pathology with severe forms of reproductive system damage, but also the influence of regional nal peculiarities on these diseases. It is emphasised that in the Republic of Tajikistan endocrine forms of infertility in women were found in the form of hypothalamic-pituitary dysfunction (polycystic ovary syndrome - 24.7%), hyperprolactinemia - 18.5%, hypothalamic-pituitary insufficiency (hypogonadotropic hypog on dysm - 2.8%), ovarian insufficiency (hypergonadotropic hypogonadism - 1.6%), congenital malformations of reproductive organs - 7.7%, hypothyroidism (Van Wyk-Ross-Henness syndrome) - 8.6% of cases. The prevalence of congenital malformations of the reproductive organs and hypothyroidism in the structure of endocr rine forms of infertility is characteristic of Tajikistan. Both in the meno- and postmenopausal period, reproductive system disorders have been recorded in Tajik women, which have regional peculiarities and are related to ethnic, climatic-geographical, socio-economic conditions of reproductive function and reproductive behaviour [74]. These peculiarities require new approaches to the prevention and diagnosis of these diseases in this contingent of patients in terms of reproductive system recovery - [101].

L.V. Sholokhov et al. [98] by comparing different ethnic groups of Tofolaria (a historical and cultural region in the central part of the

Eastern Sayan in the west of the Irkutsk region) showed that in girls of ethnic Tof and European girls already in the age group of 7-11 years there are differences in the content of active fractions of thyroid hormones, indicating different mechanisms of maintaining thyroid homeostasis. These differences persist in the age group of 12-14 years, and changes in the pituitary part of this system are added to the existing differences. Functioning of the pituitary-thyroid link of the system of neuroendocrine regulation in girls of 15-18 years old, who are indigenous inhabitants of Tofalaria, proceeds in a more economical mode. This seems to be a consequence of genetically determined long-term adaptation of the organism of indigenous people to extreme climatic and geographical environmental factors.

A scientific assessment of the peculiarities of reproductive health of adolescent girls in Mordovia is presented in the work of N.A. Buralkina [28], and of girls of different ethnic groups in Altai in the article by E.S. Vemilyaeva and E.G. Voronkov [28].

The article by E.M. Aleksandrova et al [3] presents the results of the study of obstetric pathology, fetal growth rate, morphometric indicators of women of different ethnic groups. The perspectives of ethnicity in the development of regional standards were determined.

In the work of A.V. Labygina et al. - [41] established the significance of thyroid hormone changes in infertility in different ethnic groups: for infertile and fertile Russian women living in the Republic of Buryatia, informative signs are thyroid hormone levels, for infertile and fertile Buryat women - indicators of bound thyroxine, and for European women with infertility, uterine myoma and endometriosis living in the Irkutsk region - levels of thyroxine and triiodothyronine.

L.F. Pisareva [51] studied the hormonal status of women of different nationalities (Altai, Buryat, Russian, Tuvan, Khakaski) living in Siberia and the Far East, and showed that each ethnic group is unique and has a hormonal status peculiar to it. Ethnic differences in the physical status (height and weight) of women have been revealed . It is assumed that the risk of breast cancer development is associated with an imbalance in hormonal homeostasis caused by external environmental factors. Information on the distribution of quantitative indicators of hormonal status and the systemic nature of endocrine gland reactions in indigenous Pamirians is also presented by A.V.Stepnova [28].

According to I.V.Radysh et al [28], there are significant intra-annual fertility fluctuations in all women living in the Polar region. The peculiarity of hormonal homeostasis in women of the Far North is a high percentage of additional elevations of prolactin and gonadotropins in blood plasma, especially luteinising hormone. It has been established that women in polar regions have a decrease in fertility during the polar night. In particular, menstruation cessation during this period has been described in Eskimo women.

L.M.Christian et al. - [141] in their studies showed that African-American women have twice as many premature births as white women.

F.Wakeel et al. - [226] studied the influence of racial and ethnic factors on pregnancy. Using multivariate generalised linear multivariate models, the relationship between racial and ethnic factors of Los Angeles women and pregnancy was shown.

Important factors that have an adverse effect on women and offspring include environmental influences, which are determined by the condition of the air basin, soil, the composition of drinking water and food shields, atmospheric phenomena, and solar activity [3, 9, 32, 109, 111]. The nature and quantity of food intake in certain regions is also often associated with women's reproductive health, as shown by Chinese researchers in their work on the impact of underweight and overweight on this important function ta [185]. In connection with the actively developing agriculture under market economy conditions, many new chemical preparations of different action (herbicides, fungicides, insecticides, seed dressing agents and others) are annually introduced into widespread practice to increase yields and preserve products. The mechanisms of their effects on reproduction of living organisms are actively discussed in the literature [1, 44].

The ecological and physiological features of the female organism of the indigenous inhabitants of the polar region are associated with such facts that the age of menarche in Evenk girls is 13.2 years, and in girls of the Nenets District - 12.6-13.0 years. The co ren natives of Chukotka have a later age of menarche - 13.9 years - [42].

A study by S.M. Mukhamadieva [46] of reproductive function in hot climates revealed that the average age of onset of menarche in India - in the districts of the Dakama Plateau - is 13.5 years, and in the state of Bihar - 12.9 years. For girls in Burma and Assamma it is 13.2 years, in Nigeria 14.3 years, in Syria 12.1 years, and in Tajikistan 13.5 years. According to N.B. Timofeeva (2007), in Uzbekistan, the average age of menarche for urban girls was 13.2 years, while for rural girls it was 14.4 years.

Ecological and physiological studies of indigenous populations have revealed a later onset of menarche in women living in mountainous conditions. It has been established that girls in the mountainous regions of the Caucasus have their first menses two years later than their counterparts in the plains. The same was found in the Eastern Pamir (altitude 3600-4000 metres). The later maturation of

Kyrgyz girls with heavy (47.1 per cent) and painful (44 per cent) menses has been found [42].

In the course of adaptation to specific natural, climatic and social conditions, an ecological portrait of a new ethnos is formed with a unique culture roi and peculiar morphophysiological traits, which together constitute the "body" of the ethnos, ensuring long-term preservation of biological ecial and cultural certainty and influence on reproductive health - [43, 104]. In modern conditions there is a process of ethnos degradation and it is caused by civilisation, which influences ethnoses as a powerful destructive factor - [59]. Medicine needs to change its outdated postulates, introduce new scientifically grounded paradigms, new moral and ethical principles, taking into account individual, including gender, age, ethnic peculiarities of a person. This is especially important since the problems of repro duc ulation are increasingly being solved with the help of in vitro fertilisation - [28], which requires mandatory consideration of these features. In this regard, the study of ethnic problems of adaptation of individuals living in different climatic and geographical regions seems to be relevant.

1.3 The role of genetic factors in disorders reproductive functions

The fact that chromosomal abnormalities may underlie infertility, pregnancy failure and other manifestations of reproductive disorders is beyond doubt [4, 37, 120, 124].

Many researchers believe that fetal losses are most often immunological in nature, and therefore HLA-antigens (HLA - human leukocyte antygenes) play a special role in reproductive failures [144, 146, 228]. They are located on the surface of all cells and control the immune response, which means that they play an important role in the course of the gestational process. HLA antigens are glycoproteins (a complex of proteins and carbohydrates), the composition of each of which is encoded by the corresponding HLA-gene of the 6th chromosome. In other words, the individual combination of HLA-antigens in a particular person is determined by the individual combination of HLA-genes. Each of the genes can have many dozens of variants (alleles) - their various combinations form the above-mentioned set of gene combinations. There are 2 classes of HLA antigens. Class I includes antigens of loci A, B and C, and class II includes antigens of loci DR, DP and DQ. Class I antigens are present on the surface of all nuclear cells of the human body (as well as platelets), class II antigens - on the surface of nos of cells involved in immunological reactions (B-lymphocytes, activated T-lymphocytes, monocytes, macrophages and dendritic cells) - [13, 50, 69].

Shared HLA antigens have been found to be more common in couples with non-pregnancy than in couples with normal pregnancies [31, 97]. In particular, the risk of reproductive duc dysfunction is increased in couples where the potential father has HLA-B13 and/or DQB1*0501 antigens in his phenotype (57).

The immunological hy relationship between the embryo and the mother's body influences the course and outcome of pregnancy. The maternal organism can produce antibodies to the antigens of the embryo's main histo compatibility complex, which causes immune incompatibility reactions between the maternal organism and the embryo during implantation, which can result in pregnancy failure. In this regard, the degree of HLA allele compatibility between spouses may affect the course of pregnancy, and complete incompatibility of

HLA genotypes, especially class II, is a favourable factor for the development of pregnancy - [11, 57].

O.N.Bespalova et al. [28], X.P.Wang, Q.D.Lin [28] showed that some alleles of the studied HLA class II genes are protective (alleles DRB1*15, DQA1*101, DQA1*102, DQA1*201) in terms of pregnancy development, while others may predispose to both single (spontaneous) and habitual pregnancy failure (alleles DRB1*04, DQA1*103, DQA1*301 and DQB1*302).

Certain alleles of HLA class II genes are not only associated with foetal failure but also with serious complications of pregnancy - [123, 177]. For example, an association study between specific HLA class Ia (HLA-A and -B) and class II (HLA-DRB1, - DQA1, -DQB1, - DPA1 and - DPB1) alleles found that, for example, the HLA-DPB1*04: allele was significantly more common among women with severe pre-eclampsia/eclampsia - [169].

Not only the polymorphic structure of class II HLA genes plays an important role in women's reproductive health. In recent years, class I HLA-antigens have attracted increasing attention in terms of their association with the fulfilment of reproductive functions - [5].

In this regard, one can agree with the arguments put forward by F.Grimstad, S.Krieg [159], according to which studies in recent years have shown that most often these causes of sporadic and habitual pregnancy failure are immunogenetic in nature and are associated with abnormal reactions of natural killer cells and endometrial T-cells as lymphocytes of innate and adaptive immune response. It is in this connection that allelic variants of genes responsible for the synthesis of human leukocyte antigen (HLA) class I and cytokines are being studied, and promising results have been obtained, although so far they are not so numerous as to significantly influence the current state of the art in reproductive immunogenetics - [73, 180].

There is another aspect related to the immunogenetics of reproduction. Cells of the immune system with cytotoxic activity carry receptors on their membranes that can recognise HLA class I molecules and, through the received signal, inhibit bi or activate these cells. Among such receptors are KIR - Killing Immunoglobulin Receptors, and KLR - Killing Lectin Receptors [88, 183, 207]. For example, KIRs, according to a number of researchers va , contribute to two functions in the organism - defence against infectious agents (KIR A) and reproductive success (KIR B) by participating in the restriction of trophoblast ingrowth [28] and formation of the placental vascular network [28].

The role of KLR ligands in the realisation of rep roduct ive health has been characterised in more detail. In particular, the HLA-G molecule belongs to the category of non-classical HLA class Ib, determines immune tolerance, is recognised by natural killer cells and T-lymphocytes via KIR/KLR and therefore plays an important role in maintaining successful pregnancy and maternal resistance to semi-allogeneic fetal antigens. It was shown that certain alleles of the HLA-G gene (14bp) were significantly less frequent in women with habitual pregnancy failure, which suggests the importance of this polymorphism for the realisation of reproductive function in women [112, 170]. HLA-MICB molecules are stress-induced, have population-specific expression patterns, and are associated with reproductive health [19].

The role of gene polymorphisms and other non-classical histo sov class I molecules in the development of early pregnancy failure - HLA-E and HLA-F - has been described [155].

There is another group of molecules in the HLA system - class III molecules, which include, in particular, tumour necrosis factor α (TNFα). It has been established that one of the mechanisms of predisposition to habitual miscarriage may be due to hypersecretion of TNFα at the fetal-maternal tissue interface [95], but this side of the immunogenetics of reproduction is still poorly understood.

The study of the role of immunogenetic factors in disorders of reproductive processes in a couple is one of the most demanded methods of diagnosing infertility. At present, infertility and pregnancy failure are considered as multifactorial diseases va resulting from the combined influence of genetic and environmental factors, the role of which is different for each clinical case - [57], and our understanding of the role of genetic factors in the formation of reproductive health is constantly expanding.

1.4 Role of endocrine factors in disorders reproductive function in women

The last decades of the past century are characterised by significant achievements in the field of diagnostics and treatment of various forms of fertility disorders. Traditionally and quite justifiably, endocrine factors are singled out in the structure of reproductive disorders - [28, 49, 190], because in the general system of neuro-hormonal regulation of the organism reproductive hormones, possessing a wide spectrum of action, high biological activity, pronounced metabolic effect, are given a special place - [120, 152]. The possibility of adequate adaptation of a woman's organism to the environment is largely ensured by the influence of sex hormones, changes in the concentration of which lead to significant differences in the humoral regulation of body functions - [23, 49, 28].

Such CNS structures as the hypothalamus and pituitary gland, which produce gonadotropic hormones: luteinising and follicle mulating hormones, as well as prolactin, are directly involved in many physiological processes, including morphogenesis, specific cellular functions, and reproductive behaviour in general and the gestational process in particular - [84].

The next structural link of the reproductive system is the ovary, which fulfils two important functions in the female organism: reproductive, expressed in the formation of female germ cells, and endocrine, realised in the production of sex hormones - mainly estrogens and progesterone, as well as their main source - androgens - [39]. The ovary functions cyclically and, therefore, its structure and endocrine production depend on the phase of the menstrual (ovarian) cycle or the presence of pregnancy [25, 58, 77].

Speaking about the cyclic nature of hormonal restructuring in the female organism, the following algorithm should be emphasised. Follicle-stimulating hormone (FSH), or follitropin, is produced by the pituitary gland and causes the growth and maturation of ovarian follicles, their preparation for ovulation - [82]. The most important regulator of FSH in the female organism is antimüllerian hormone (AMH), produced by special granulosa cells of growing follicles and currently used to determine the ovarian reserve of women - [16, 82, 137,

160], and follicular redox balance may be important for the quality of embryos during in vitro fertilisation (IVF) - [196].

Under the influence of follicle-stimulating hormone in the ovaries, the growth of follicles with a size from 2 to 10 mm is significantly accelerated, which takes about 7 days - [151]. Next, the dominant follicle is selected, which has receptors for luteinising hormone and begins to produce estradiol into the blood - [12, 175].

While the biological action of FSH is directly directed at folliculogenesis, the effect of luteinising hormone (LH) on follicle development is related to its ability to modulate the production of sex steroids (steroidogenesis) - [226].

Thus, under the influence of luteinising hormone, androgens are formed from cholesterol in the theca cells of the ovary. Androgens from theca-cells get into granulosa cells (cells of the granular layer of follicular epithelium), where under the action of follicle-stimulating hormone on the aromatase enzyme complex are converted into estrogens, in particular, testosterone is converted into estradiol - [67].

Testosterone is the most important androgenic and natural anabo lytic hormone in men and women - [67]. Disorders of female reproductive function are quite often observed in hyperandrogenism, a pathological condition caused by altered secretion of androgens, disturbance of their metabolism and binding in the periphery. Androgens, being direct precursors of female sex hormones, are necessary in the development of reproductive ive function and maintenance of hormonal homeostasis. Violation of biosynthesis and metabolism of androgens has a long-term, persistent effect on various parts of the reproductive system of the female body. In this case, the increased level of testosterone in women may be of adrenal or ovarian origin, and to identify the cause of hyperandrogenism helps diagnostic determination of the level of dehydroepiandrosterone, which is synthesised mainly by the adrenal cortex and only partially by the sex glands. Hyperandrogenism in women is often called the disease of the century and is associated with scientific and technological progress, increased mental and physical activity, urbanisation, and the influence of stressful situations [90, 91].

Estradiol is the main estrogen that functions from puberty to menopause; it is responsible for more than four hundred functions in the female body. In addition to the ovaries, estradiol can also be produced in small amounts in the reticular zone of the adrenal cortex . Many researchers consider excessive estro genes to be a possible cause of endometrial and breast cancer, especially in obese women - [67].

As the dominant follicle forms and estradiol production increases, FSH levels decrease and, as a consequence, the other (non-leading) follicles develop in reverse, and the leading follicle changes from an FSH-dependent to an LH/FSH-dependent stage. As the dominant follicle develops, it fills with follicular fluid containing estradiol in particular and pushes the ovum towards one of the poles, turning the follicle into a Graaff bubble - [26]. This whole mechanism is included in the concept of "two-cell theory of steroidogenesis" - [91, 175]. Ovulation is the culmination of neurohumoral processes that ensure the cyclic functions of the reproductive system - [25].

During ovulation, the follicle bursts and the ovum is sent into the fallopian tube, while the former follicle is replaced by the corpus luteum, which is an important endocrine formation that produces another hormone, progesterone. This leads to a significant increase in the amount of progesterone in the body, the level of which reaches a maximum about 7 days before the onset of menstruation - [22, 28].

Progesterone is not only one of the steroid hormones, but is practically the progenitor of the vast majority of them [67]. The primary function of progesterone is to support pregnancy, since its biological role is to prepare the estrogen-stimulated endometrium for implantation of a fertilised egg [54, 55, 28].

Progesterone receptors (two types) are found not only in endometrium, myometrium, preovulatory and luteinised granulosa cells, corpus luteum, testes, mammary glands, but also in endothelium, thymus, osteoblasts, bronchi, lungs, pancreas. The receptor defect results in the absence of endometrial changes characteristic of the secretory phase of the menstrual cycle. Complete receptor resistance is accompanied by female infertility, partial receptor resistance is accompanied by possible infertility and spontaneous miscarriages [67].

As for the corpus luteum as the main producer of progesterone, if the ovum has not been fertilised, the corpus luteum still functions for 12-15 days. At the end of this period, it dies and the woman menstruates - [39].

When the ovum is fertilised, the corpus luteum, as already mentioned, contributes to pregnancy. In this case, it remains active for 13-15 weeks from the moment of fertilisation. After the 15th week, the corpus luteum transfers its "powers" to the placenta. At this point, the corpus luteum ceases its activity and a barely visible scar is formed in its place [82, 84].

The process of implantation of a fertilised oocyte as such, as well as paracrine and autocrine regulation of this process initiated by implantation, requires some attention [131, 161, 202, 28]. The implantation process proceeds in several stages: (1) unstable adhesion of the fertilised voren oocyte (blastocyst) to the functional layer of the endometrium (decis dual sheath), (2) stable adhesion, (3) invasion stage with the formation of trophoblast with subsequent processes of angiogenesis - [142, 220, 28]. During the stage of stable adhesion a very important role belongs to adhesion molecules - E-cadherins of blastocyst villi (pinopods) - [220] and integrins of the decidual membrane - [135, 211, 28], regulated by estradiol - [157], as well as uterine glycoproteins MUC1, the expression of which is regulated by progeste ron - [162, 28]. Growth factors - epidermal growth factor - [212, 229, 28], tumour necrosis factor α produced by both trophoblast and endometrial cells - [28] and others are of great importance in the implantation process for the development of both trophoblast and decidual membrane through the proliferative activity of cells. The most important functional significance in the realisation of all these processes belongs, first of all, to progesterone [156, 165, 167, 178, 28].

Returning to the regulatory role of sex hormones, it may be added that in women of childbearing age, the secretion of gonadotropins plays a very important role in the regulation of the menstrual cycle. During menopause, the production of sex hormones decreases and, due to negative feedback, the secretion of gonadotropins by the pituitary gland (in particular, FSH) increases significantly, proving to be higher than in the childbearing period [14, 24, 53, 105]. Low levels of gonadotropins can be observed, for example, in hypophy zar insufficiency - [53, 105, 222]. In the case of delayed sexual development, the diagnosis of hormonal disorders in girls follows the pattern corresponding to the detection of ovarian insufficiency. An elevated FSH level in the blood is the basis for a complete endocrinological and genetic examination. In cases of early puberty, the concentration of gonadotropins in the blood is elevated compared to the normal level for this age (53).

In the anterior lobe of the pituitary gland, lactotrophic cells synthesise another hormone important for the realisation of reproductive function - prolactin. The number of these lactotrophic cells increases dramatically during pregnancy under the influence of estrogen. Prolactin is one of the most ancient hormones of the pituitary gland, as it is found, except in mammals, in animals without lactation systems - [56, 98, 126]. Prolactin receptors are present in cells of many tissues: in the liver, kidneys, adrenal glands, testes, ovaries, uterus and other tissues. The main function of prolactin is to stimulate lactation; in addition, since it is somewhat similar in structure to growth hormone, it may have a similar effect on the organism, although to a somewhat lesser extent [66].

Both hyperprolactinaemia and hypoprolactinaemia have been found to contribute to reproductive dysfunction and often serve as a cause of infertility not only in women but also in men - [163, 230].

The hypothalamic-pituitary-ovarian and hypothalamic-pituitary-thyroid systems are closely linked, which is realised due to the presence of common central mechanisms of regulation. . The functions of the sexual and thyroid systems are regulated by tropic hormones of the anterior lobe of the pituitary gland. The thyrotropin-releasing hormone (thyroliberin) of the hypothalamus is a stimulant not only of thyroid hormone (TTH), but also of pituitary prolactin, so dysfunction of the pituitary-thyroid system leads to changes not only in gonadotropins, but also in prolactin - [67].

Indeed, the most common endocrine pathology in women of reproductive age is thyroid disease [79, 99]. Thyroid pathology may be the cause of premature or late puberty, menstrual disorders, infertility, galactorrhoea, pregnancy failure, fetal and neonatal pathology. In turn, the state of the reproductive system has a significant impact on thyroid function. This is confirmed by changes in thyroid function during pregnancy and lactation in patients with benign tumours and hyperplastic processes of the female genital organs. It is now proved that estrogens have a pronounced stimulating effect on the thyroid gland, primarily due to the intensification of thyroxine-binding globulin synthesis in the liver. In addition, estrogens increase the sensitivity of pituitary thyrotrophs to thyrolyl berin. On the contrary, under conditions of prolonged hypoestrogenism, the sensitivity of thyrotrophs to thyroliberin decreases, which can be considered as one of the possible mechanisms for the development of secondary hypothyroidism in women with hypoestrogenic conditions [79, 92, 99].

Experimental work in recent decades has provided evidence for the presence of receptors for thyroid hormone and triiodothyronine in the ovary and thus a direct influence of thyroid dys function on steroidogenesis and oocyte maturation. Thyroid hormones act unidirectionally with follicle-stimulating hormone, having a direct sti muli effect on the function of granulosa cells (including their morphological gical differentiation), stimulate progesterone and estradiol secretion; they influence the fertilisation capacity of oocytes, the quality and viability of embryos - [79, 100].

Various reproductive disorders in women are often accompanied by changes in adrenal function, which are manifested by increased blood levels of steroids such as cortisol and 17-hydroxyprogesterone as an intermediate product of steroid synthesis in the adrenal cortex and gonads [72].

In clinical practice, isolated disorders of endocrine glands are almost never encountered. Usually there is a predominant disorder of the functions of one gland in combination with more or less pronounced disorders of other associated functions. This is a consequence of the interaction of hormones among themselves, which can be manifested already at the level of their synthesis. In this regard, the study of hormones should be carried out comprehensively, taking into account their permissive action [53, 92, 99, 108].

1.5 The role of the immune system in disordered behaviour reproductive function in women

It is now known that about 80% of previously unexplained recurrent pregnancy losses are associated with unrecognised immunological disorders - [207].

An important method of examination in patients with impaired reproductive function is the study of immune status, since the immune system of the female reproductive tract, according to S.K. Lee et al. - [184] has two main functions: defence against microbes and preservation of pregnancy for a defined period.

The study of the immunology of the reproductive process occurring in the female organism has advanced considerably in recent years [27, 225, 90], with all three major lymphocyte populations - B cells, T cells, and natural killer cells - being characterised in detail in pregnancy and reproductive disorders, and the endometrium being the main biotope where all major molecular [28; 90] and cellular - [90] immunological processes, as well as structural and functional changes

- [227, 90], is the endometrium - [200]. A very important function in this biotope belongs to various cytokines of the immune system, such as epidermal growth factor in the implantation of the fertilised egg - [90], tumour necrosis factor α - [127, 129, 141], interleukin-1 - [191, 90], interleukin-6 and its receptor on the endometrium gp130 - [150, 28], interleukin-10 - [221], chemokines - [182].

Immunophenotyping of peripheral blood lymphocytes and assessment of the presence of immunocompetent cells in tissues allows us to identify abnormalities and determine the quantitative composition of cells responsible for the production of proinflammatory cytokines and autoantibodies [90].

Natural killer cells (NK, NK, CD16+CD56+), being lymphocytes of innate immunity, play an important role in immune defence mechanisms and contribute to either reproductive success or pregnancy failure - [214, 231, 90], as evidenced by the correspondence of an increase in the content of NK in the blood of women to the development of reproductive disorders - [145, 168, 192].

This is due to the ability of ECs to express on their surface a special category of receptors - inhibitory and activating receptors, the ligands for which are HLA class I molecules. Most of the receptors are of immuno globulin nature (KIR) and are identified on the EC surface using markers CD158a-z. The ligands for these receptors are more often the classical [HLA-A,B,C] class I histocompatibility molecules, although in isolated cases KIRs can interact with some non-classical class I histocompatibility molecules, such as HLA-G. In addition to KIRs, ECs have inhibitory and activating lectin receptors (KLRs), the main ligands for which are non-classical class I histocompatibility molecules, as well as stress-induced cellular molecules. Thus, inhibitory receptors of ECs take predominant part in interaction with classical class I NLAs on the surface of healthy cells, so healthy cells are not exposed to cytotoxic influence of ECs. If the cell is foreign (carries allogeneic HLA molecules), or is damaged by a pathological process, or is stress-induced, it will cause an attack of natural killer cells through the effect on activating receptors [88, 110, 22].

Natural killer cells are very widely represented at the site of maternal-fetal contact, where, in early pregnancy, fetal trophoblast cells characterised by marked expression of HLA-G (non-classical class I histocompatibility molecules) are present - [88, 153, 28]. As the placenta begins to form, the expression of HLA-C (classical class I histocompatibility molecules) begins to predominate [149, 90]. ECs in the decidual uterine lining account for about 20-30% of the number of cells of medullary origin, where they limit trophoblast ingrowth and control the development of the placenta - [110, 198].

Soluble HLA-G interacts with KIR - immunoglobulin-activated activating natural killer receptors CD158d, which initiate signalling pathways of pro-inflammatory and pro-angiogenic reactions. As a result of constant activation of CD158d, ECs show morphological changes , which indicate the aging of these cells and the formation of a secretory (rather than cytotoxic) phenotype. The secretory phenotype programme is usually implemented in response to oncogenes or DNA damage, and the secretory products secreted help to limit cell growth and tissue repair. In the uterus of pregnant women, secretory products induced by signalling systems from CD158d stimulate vascular remodelling and angiogenesis through the formation of endothelial cell tubes, i.e. they play an essential role in placental development in early pregnancy [271]. There is evidence of the role of KIR-haplotype in reproductive disorders in women [116, 221, 28].

As the placenta forms, it has been indicated that HLA-C expression begins to predominate, serving as an inducer of predominantly inhibitory signals, and some alleles of genes responsible for the interaction of these molecules with the KIR of natural killer cells may combine with disruption of the placental barrier and inhibit fetal growth - [149].

There is also evidence that the expression of KIR and KLR in the uterus outside of pregnancy is dependent on the phase of the menstrual cycle [193], although the question of the biological significance of this phenomenon has not yet been resolved.

There is evidence of a similar mechanism of regulation involving inhibitory and activating lectin receptors (KLR) in Tγδ-lymphocytes [119], also inhabiting the decidual membrane.

In addition to ECs and Tγδ, another category of innate immunity lymphocytes, ECT (CD3+CD56+), is elevated in the uterine mucosa [110, 145, 176]. These cells populating the mucous membranes have a very pronounced regulatory effect through the production of cytokines and, depending on their subpopulation, can regulate the ratio of type 1 and type 2 T-helper cells (i.e., the ratio of cellular and humoral reactions), and can have an immunosuppressive effect - [89].

Among the cells of innate immunity, macrophages of the uterine decidual membrane play a certain role in the formation of the placenta. Among them 2 phenotypes are distinguished - CD11c high (20%) and CD11c low (68%). CD11c high expression is associated with lipid metabolism, inflammation, fetal antigen presentation, while CD11c low macrophages are associated with extracellular matrix formation, regulation of muscle tissue and cell growth in the process of placenta formation - [188].

As for the involvement of T-lymphocytes in immune processes related to reproduction, prolactin plays a very important role. This hormone acts as a cytokine in contact with immune system cells. In particular, the analysis of intracellular signalling pathways in the process of activation of IL-2 genes as T-cell growth factor and prolactin suggests that the action of these two cytokines is highly coordinated when they simultaneously act on T-lymphocyte receptors [90].

The content of T-lymphocytes in the decidual membrane is quite high in the initial period after its formation, although somewhat lower than ECs, but by the end of pregnancy their number decreases to 5-8% of the total number of leukocytes. T cells of this localisation include both CD4+ (T-helper cells) and CD8+ (cytotoxic T-lymphocytes, CTL). Interestingly, during pregnancy , type 1 T-helpers slightly predominate in the decidual membrane, while type 2 T-helpers predominate in the blood [110].

The scientific literature discusses the role of type 17 T-helper cells in women's reproductive health disorders. These cells produce cyto kines of pronounced proinflammatory action. It has been reported that the content of Tx17 cells is significantly increased in the decidual membrane of women with non-pregnancy - [28, 90]. However, this has been shown to occur only in the presence of haemorrhage - [28], and it has been suggested that the increase in Tx17 is a consequence rather than a cause of miscarriage - [90].

It is known that during gestation, maternal T-lymphocytes are involved in immune reactions directed against paternal alloantigens present in the foetus. In this connection, cells with immuno suppress activity gradually begin to play an increasing role in the composition of the uterine decidual membrane during pregnancy, which is the main mechanism for ensuring immunological tolerance of the mother to semi-allogeneic antigenic structures of the foetus. The largest proportion of regulatory T cells (Treg, CD3+CD4+CD25+FoxP3+) are [117, 176, 181, 206] - lymphocytes of thymic or peripheral origin, the main function of which is to secrete cytokines of immunosuppressive action - transforming growth factor β (TGFβ), IL-35, IL-10, etc. [110, 117]. - [110, 117]. Judging by experimental data, the importance of Treg in the development of maternal immunotolerance to the foetus is formed rather early, because the introduction of these cells into experimental animals immediately before the development of pregnancy promotes the increase in the levels of cytokines of these cells - TFRβ and IL-10, and after the onset of pregnancy has no effect [90]. It has also been shown that the deficiency of Tregs formed from T-lymphocytes of other subpopulations (so-called inducible T-regs) in women tends to cause spontaneous miscarriages in early pregnancy [121].

In addition to Treg, regulatory B-lymphocytes (Breg), which secrete a suppressor cytokine such as IL-10, are also involved in the process of immunosuppression in pregnancy [176].

It has been established that gonadotropins, progesterone, and estradiol are involved in the formation of a pool of regulatory T- and B-cells, i.e., in the development of immune tolerance of the mother's body to fetal antigens, if they act in physiological concentrations. This effect is not realised if the level of sex hormones exceeds the physiological norm - [174].

Thus, the development of pregnancy during the realisation of reproductive function requires tolerance of the female organism to genetically foreign paternal antigens of the developing foetus. One of the main evolutionarily fixed mechanisms of such immunotolerance is a systemic increase in the proportion of the cellular population of maternal regulatory T cells (FohP3+) specific to fetal antigens. A decrease or absence of this effect is associated with the development of complications such as eclampsia, premature labour, and spontaneous pregnancy failure [143, 171, 194].

However, the fate of these regulatory T cells after delivery is unclear. Do they disappear after birth and are they generated de novo with each pregnancy or are they maintained over a long period of time? If they persist, do they contribute to the fulfilment of reproductive function later in life and do they cause any harm to the woman's body?

It is now known that maternal antigen-specific CD4+ T cells persist at elevated levels for the first 100 days after birth, and then the level of maternal Tregs of this specificity gradually decreases after delivery. In subsequent pregnancies, the pool of regulatory cells becomes even larger than in the initial pregnancy. These observations suggest that memory regulatory cells may be formed - [28]. A very important conclusion from these data is that the more often a woman develops pregnancies, the better her reproductive function is realised.

As for the role of B-lymphocytes in the realisation of reproductive function, it is related to the production of antibodies by these cells and is interpreted rather ambiguously, since B cells play a certain role both in the formation of immune tolerance and in pregnancy pathology [28], B1-lymphocytes as lymphocytes of mucous membranes and their secretory products - immunoglobulins, which have multiple specificity and can therefore participate in interaction with autoantigens - [110].

It is believed that it is the increase in the level of B1-lymphocytes in combination with an increase in the number of natural killer cells, carrying out reactions of antibody vissible cytotoxicity, that is the decisive factor in triggering reactions associated with placental abruption and pregnancy failure, in particular, in autoimmune processes in the thyroid gland - [177].

The ratio of blood immunoglobulin fractions (IgG, IgM, IgA) produced by B-lymphocytes, as well as phagocytosis indices, which are largely related to antibody formation, can also indicate possible disorders in the course of immune processes in the patient's organism [28, 121]. At the same time, most modern studies consider the participation of B-lymphocytes and the immunoglobulins of different classes (IgM, IgG, IgA, IgE) produced by them in the pathogenesis of reproductive disorders primarily from the perspective of their role in autoimmune processes, often associated with gestation [148, 28].

1.6 Autoimmune processes and disorders reproductive function in women

As follows from the data presented above, reproductive disorders in women are quite often of immune nature, with one of the most important mechanisms of pregnancy failure being associated with a breakdown of immune tolerance to foetal antigens due to genetically determined or phenotypically determined deficiency of the T- and B-regulatory cell system. Against this background, conditions are created for the development of an autoimmune process, manifestations of which include an increase in the level of EC cells and B1-lymphocytes, and a disturbance in the ratio of T-helper cells of type 1 and type 2 [158, 205].

The relationship between autoimmune diseases and reproduction appears to be bidirectional: on the one hand, autoimmune diseases can can negatively affect women of reproductive age, and, conversely, pregnancy men can affect the manifestations of autoimmune diseases.

Thus. Autoimm mune diseases not only increase the risk of miscarriage but also decrease female fertility in general, as does the success of treatment for non fetal disease. At the same time, pregnancy can have an impact on improving the course of an autoimmune disease or worsening it. During pregnancy, many autoimmune diseases go into remission only to flare up again in the early postpartum period - [177, 28, 90].

It has been observed that approximately 20% of women with habitual miscarriage have autoimmune disorders caused by antiphospholipid antibodies. In addition, the presence of antinuclear antibodies, as well as antibodies to thyroid components - thyroperoxidase and thyroglobulin - is often high in women with reproductive abnormalities [36, 114, 204, 205].

Autoimmune thyroiditis has important consequences for conception, the occurrence of pregnancy complications and the outcome of pregnancy. In addition, autoimmune mun thyroiditis can exacerbate the postpartum period and adversely affect the outcome of in vitro fertilisation - [197]. Finally, the consequences of autoimmune thyroiditis may have important implications for offspring. A.F.Muller, A.Berghout - [194] showed the association between autoimmune hypo- and hyperfunction during pregnancy and obstetric complications. After obstetric thyroiditis, according to the authors, is associated with the presence of autoantibodies to thyroperoxidase, that is, it is an autoimmune thyroiditis.

In the course of research scientists were able to reliably show the connection between the level of autoantibodies to thyroperoxidase and the presence of female infertility. Thyroid dysfunction in the presence of thyroperoxidase antibodies is a prerequisite for ovarian dysfunction. In women with this autoimmune manifestation, first of all, there is a decrease in the level of free thyroxine, which in pregnancy is accompanied by dysfunction of the urogenital tract, impaired fetal development and the risk of spontaneous abortion - [28]. In autoimmune thyroiditis, the production of IL-4 and IL-10, cytokines so important for the gestational process, is significantly reduced in the endometrium by T cells, and polyclonal B-lymphocytes without organ specificity are induced, which may impair the immunotolerance associated with pregnancy [213, 28, 90]. Clinical practice confirms that a simultaneous multiple increase in the level of antibodies to thyroperoxidase and thyroglobulin in pregnant women was quite often accompanied by premature labour and pregnancy failure - [132].

According to K. Rorre et al. - [28], autoimmune thyroiditis may not affect normal embryo implantation, but the risk of early reproductive losses is significantly increased. At the same time, J.Bellver et al. - [28] under confirmed the high prevalence of thyroid autoantibodies in reproductive disorders .

Antiphospholipid syndrome is even more widespread as a cause of reproductive dysfunction in women [71, 125, 140, 203, 28].

Antiphospholipid syndrome is an autoimmune condition of hyper coa gulation that is associated with antiphospholipid antibodies - [28].

According to modern concepts, the basis of antiphospholipid syndrome rum is the formation of autoantibodies in the organism in high titre, interacting mo with negatively charged plasma phospholipid membranes and associated proteins-glycoproteins. The main mi she n ns of antiphospholipid antibodies are negatively charged cardio lipin, phosphatidylserine, phosphatidylethanolamine, and phosphatidylic acid, and the protein components are β2glycoprotein-I, annexin V, and prothrombin [35, 75, 28].

Antibodies involved in the pathogenesis of antiphospholipid syndrome predict tav is a family of heterogeneous auto- and alloimmune immunoglobulins belonging to different classes: IgG, IgA, IgM - [94, 28].

The relationship between autoantibodies of different specificity and the pathogenesis of antiphospholipid syndrome is not uniform. Thus, IgG-antibodies to β2-glycoprotein-1, more specifically, autoantibodies to the first domain of this protein - [118, 159], as they provoke fetal loss due to stimulation of thrombosis - [113], play a major role in the development of patho lo gy of pregnancy.

IgG-autoantibodies to prothrombin are also closely related to the manifestations of antiphospholipid syndrome [130, 28, 90]. The diagnostic significance of these autoantibodies in the recognition of antiphospholipid syndrome is particularly high when anti-β2-glycoprotein-1 and lupus antioagulant are detected in parallel with them [28].

Antiphospholipid antibodies, which include the so-called anti-cardiolipin antibodies and lupus anticoagulant, are a group of heterogeneous antibodies that bind phospholipid-protein comp lexes. Much more often autoantibodies to phospholipids (APA) are determined, which include total antibodies to cardiolipin, phosphatidylserine, phosphatidyl linositol, phosphatidyl acid. At the same time, in clinical practice, immunoenzymatic determination of antibodies to cardiolipin, which is the main fraction of AFA, serves as one of the most valuable and standardised tests for the diagnosis of antiphospholipid syndrome - [85, 215].

The presence of autoantibodies to annexin V is also of some importance in the diagnosis of antiphospholipid syndrome. Annexins are a family of 12 proteins capable of calcium-dependent interaction with phospholipids [28], and annexin V competes with coagulation factors, disrupting blood coagulation processes [134]. Since annexin is expressed by the placenta in a rather large amount - [136], the presence of antibodies to it in a woman's organism will promote thrombosis in the placental tissue - [90].

The presence of a set of autoantibodies against phospholipids called lupus anticoagulant can be detected by prolongation of blood clotting time using a variety of tests [28], and its detection in blood is a qualitative manifestation of the action of certain levels of autoantibodies to phospholipids on the haemostasis system [87, 172].

The pathogenesis of antiphospholipid syndrome is as follows. Thrombosis, a key factor in the disease, can result from a variety of mechanisms, including the involvement of endothelial cells, monocytes, platelets, components of the coagulation system, and blockage of the fibrino lytic and anti-coagulation pathways. The trigger is the binding of antiphospholipid antibodies to receptors on target cells, causing their activation and leading to thrombosis in large vessels - [164]. The receptors attaching such autoantibodies are extremely diverse in their composition. They include annexin A2 on endothelial cells - [224, 28], apolipoprotein E receptor 2 on monocytes, endothelium, trophoblast cells - [28], receptor to low-density lipoproteins - [90] and megalin [28] on endothelial cells, Toll-like receptors 2 and 4 on monocytes and endothelial cells - [115, 28]. It has also been shown that β2-glycoprotein-1 can reside on the surface of platelets and attach appropriate antibodies - [90]. The result of all these interactions is vascular hyperplasia with the development of chronic vasculopathy with disturbances of blood coagulation processes - [138].

Antiphospholipid syndrome is manifested by arterial or venous thrombosis in vessels of various calibres and is very closely associated with repro duction disorders - [130, 133] and pregnancy complications in the form of pre-eclampsia/eclampsia - [216, 90]. According to M. Sugiura-Ogasawara et al. [90], the cause of miscarriage of pregnancy at a later stage in the progression of antiphospholipid syndrome is the development of thrombotic vasculopathy of the spiral arteries of the placenta. In addition to pregnancy pathology, the syndrome is characterised by gangrene and ulcers of the extremities, organ infarcts, neurological symptomatology (strokes, multiple sclerosis, seizure syndrome), some psychiatric diseases and other symptoms, blood clotting disorders. As a result, the risk of microthrombosis is increased, and in pregnant women the formation of the placenta is disturbed and miscarriage occurs - [122].

Anticardiolipin antibodies, anti-β2-glycoprotein 1 and lupus anticoagulant, as mentioned, are the main groups of autoantibodies that are definitive for the development of this syndrome - [28]. In singleton pregnancies with primary antiphospholipid syndrome, anticardiolipin antibodies are the most common sign of antiphospholipid syndrome - [90]. At the same time, antibodies to β2-glycoprotein I served as the main sign associated with a low birth rate, a high incidence of pre-eclampsia, intrauterine fetal growth restriction and stillbirth compared with the presence of anticardiolipin antibodies or lupus anticoagulant alone. If all three signs are registered, then, according to G. Saccone et al. - [28], despite therapy, the chance of successful completion of pregnancy is only 30%.

In recent years, many researchers have focused their efforts on developing methods for quantifying the risk of thrombosis and fetal loss in antiphospholipid syndrome [130, 28]. For this purpose, scales are proposed, the calculation of which is based on a combination of various laboratory signs of antiphospholipid syndrome. Examples are the scales introduced, in particular, in the United Kingdom (UK), such as, for example, the aPL-S scale, which includes 6 indicators based on autoantibodies (IgG/IgM antibodies to cardiolipin, IgG/IgM antibodies to β2-glycoprotein-1, IgG/IgM antibodies to phospholipids/prothrombin) and 5 indicators of lupus anticoagulant determination - [28, 90], as well as the GAPSS scale based on 16 indicators - [90].

Summary to chapter 1

1 The protection of women's reproductive health is one of the most important medical and social problems of state importance, since women's reproductive health is the main potential for reproduction of the country's population, its demographic resource, without which neither economic nor social growth of the state is possible.

2. Both physiological indicators of reproductive health and the nature of its disorders depend on the climatic, geographical and

environmental conditions in which a woman lives and her ethnicity.

3 The study of the role of immunogenetic factors in reproductive disorders is extremely promising from the point of view of the prognosis of reproductive disorders and the fight against infertility, but this aspect of the study of the problem is still far from the final disclosure of the role of immunogenetics in the formation of reproductive health.

4. The importance of hormonal status in the formation of reproductive health is beyond doubt and is being intensively studied, with the population features of hormonal support of reproductive functions remaining one of the topical areas of research.

5. Reproductive immunology, on the one hand, requires in-depth interpretation of immunological mechanisms, and on the other hand, needs reliable markers of immunopathological conditions associated with reproductive disorders.

6. The frequency of the combination of autoimmune pathology and reproductive disorders needs to be assessed from a population perspective.

7. All causes and conditions of reproductive health disorders are closely related and are usually realised in complex combinations with each other.

8. The example of antiphospholipid syndrome shows the prospect of developing scales for quantitative risk assessment of reproductive health disorders, which would make it possible to start creating and widely implementing a system of effective measures for their prevention.

CHAPTER 2. MATERIALS AND METHODS OF RESEARCH

2.1 Objects of the study

The work was carried out within the framework of the CIS International Scientific Research conducted by the Federal State Budgetary Educational Institution of Higher Education "Lipetsk State Pedagogical University sytet", Department of Biomedical Disciplines, Lipetsk, Russia, and the Tajik State Medical University (Republic of Tajikistan).

A group of clinically healthy women in the age range of 20 to 43 years was selected for this study. From 2010 to 2015 inclusive, 1,025 women were examined - 515 women living in Lipetsk Oblast (Russia) and 510 women living in Faizabad (Republic of Tajikistan).

According to the modern classification of age categories, the age range of 15-49 years is estimated as the fertile age in women - [23]. Within this rather wide age range, in turn, there are several ring categories: (1) women in the age of early reproductive activity - 15-19 years old; (2) women in the age of highest reproductive activity - 20-34 years old; (3) women in the age of fading reproductive activity - 35-44 years old; (4) women in the age of late reproductive activity - 45-49 years old - [96]. Taking into account the fact that the main contingent of the study population should be formed from women who have given birth, the present study included women of two age categories - the second and third, i.e. from 20 to 44 years of age.

Thus, all women under observation were of fertile age - from 20 to 44 years, their average age was 28.1± 0.7 years. At the same time, according to the ethnic characteristics and climatic and geographical factors of the places of residence, the surveyed women belonged to two populations - Russian and Tajik.

Venous blood was collected from all 1,025 women for HLA typing by molecular genetic analysis and to determine the range of normative values of hormonal and immune status indicators, auto immune component in each population. After specifying the reference population values, women were further selected for final formation of study groups in accordance with the inclusion and non-inclusion criteria, as well as exclusion from the study, taking into account the obstetric history.

The inclusion criteria for the study included:

1) Absence of any chronic diseases;
2) absence at the time of the study of pronounced shifts (beyond the ref rence values) in the hormonal status, immune status, auto immune component of the blood, as well as the results of general clinical laboratory tory studies of blood and urine;
3) Ages 20-44.

Criteria for non-inclusion in the study were:

1) the presence of acute diseases of any etiology in the woman at the time of the study ;
2) a woman's history of severe somatic pathology, including gynaecological diseases, endocrine pathology, immunopathological log conditions;
3) the presence of mental illness in the woman;
4) pregnancy and lactation at the time of the study.

Criteria for exclusion from the study:

1) refusal of the research (absence of informed consent) and/or non-compliance with the research programme. ;
2) somatic or other severe pathology developed during the course of the research.

In the course of the research, the blood of women in the observation groups was analysed for hormonal status, immune status, the presence of an autoimmune component, and molecular genetic analysis was performed.

2.2 Population characteristics of the study groups

One of the most important characteristics of the women in the study groups was their population characteristics, which included both different subra ses and ethnicity, and different climatic and geographical conditions of residence.

The population of Russian women included representatives of the Eastern Slavic ethnic group of Caucasoid race living in the Lipetsk region. Lipetsk Oblast is *part of the* Russian Federation, is located in the central part of the East European Plain, and is characterised by a moderately continental climate (according to the Köppen climate classification:Dsb) with warm summers and moderately cold winters. All seasons of the year are clearly defined. Average temperature pe rature January -10° C, July +19° C. Precipitation is about 500 mm per year. The vegetation eration period is 180-190 days.

The population of Tajik women contained members of the Pamir-Fergana race of the Central Asian interfluve, the easternmost sub-race of the Euro peoid race distributed in Central Asia. The women were living in Faizabad at the time of the study about . This district of the Republic of Tajikistan is an area of typical mountainous country, surrounded by mountains belonging to the highest mountain systems of Central Asia - the Tien Shan and Pamir. The district is located in the densely populated and fertile Hissar valley at an altitude of 750-930 metres above sea level. Climate of Faizabad district is subtropical sharply continental (according to the classification of climates Köppe on:Dsb), somewhat mitigated by the mountainous position of the city. Summer in Faizabad is long and hot, precipitation is very rare. The winter is relatively short, with abundant precipitation, remotely reminiscent of the Mediterranean climate.

2.3 Research Methods

2.3.1 Method of molecular genetic analysis (PCR)

DNA samples were obtained from peripheral blood lymphocytes using reagent kits and protocol for DNA isolation from various biological material by "DLAtom^{TM} DNAPrep 100" (Russia).

The distribution of HLA class I antigens (A, B, C), as well as the determination of polymorphic alleles of HLA-DRB1, HLA-DQA1, and HLA-DQB1 loci were performed using a reagent kit from DNA-Technology in accordance with the instructions for use recommended by the manufacturer.

The study of carriage of HLA class I genes and genotyping of allelic variants of HLA class II (loci DRB1, DQA1, DQB1) was carried out by modification of the polymerase chain reaction method in the form of allele-specific PCR taking into account the amplified fragment length polymorphism (ALLP) and restriction fragment length polymorphism (RFLP) using a thermocycler for nucleic acid amplification iCycler with an optical module lem iCycler iQ5 in accordance with the instructions for use, as well as on a thermo cyc ler manufactured by NPO DNA-Technology LLC DTprime using software supporting automatic data processing.

The principle of determining allelic variants taking into account restriction fragment length polymorphism is to amplify phi cy a certain genetic locus using PCR. Then the amplification product is cleaved by restriction endonucleases. This produces fragments of different sizes, which, when electrophoresed, form profiles that are different for different allelic variants of the locus.

The principle of the amplified fragment length polymorphism detection method differs from the previous method in that restriction is performed before PCR starts. The DNA of blood leukocytes is cut into fragments using a restrictase, and then PCR is performed. As a result, fragments of different sizes are formed, which, when electrophoresed, produce profiles that are different for different allelic variants of the HLA class I and class II gene locus.

The combination of the above methods allowed the identification of:

- HLA-A genes - A1, A2, A3, A9, A10, A11, A19, A28, A29;
- HLA-B genes - B5, B7, B8, B12, B13, B14, B15, B16, B17, B18, B21, B22, B27, B35, B40;
- HLA-C genes - Cw2, Cw3, Cw4, Cw5;
- DRB1*01, DRB1*04, DRB1*07, DRB1*08, DRB1*09, DRB1*11, DRB1*12, DRB1*13, DRB1*14, DRB1*15, DRB1*16, DRB1*17 allelic variants within the HLA-DRB1 gene locus;
- within the HLA-DQA1 gene locus, allelic variants DQA1*0101, DQA1*0102, DQA1*0103, DQA1*0201, DQA1*0301, DQA1*0302, DQA1*0401, DQA1*0501;
- within the HLA-DQB1 gene locus, allelic variants DQB1*7, DQB1*15, DQB1*0201, DQB1*0301, DQB1*0302, DQB1*0303, DQB1*0308, DQB1*0401-2, DQB1*050, DQB1*0501, DQB1*0502, DQB1*0503, DQB1*0601, DQB1*0602, DQB1*0602-8.

2.3.2 Methods for assessing hormonal status

In obtaining the characteristics of hormonal status, we evaluated the indicators of hypothalamic-pituitary-ovarian, thyroid, corticosteroid systems in women of different ethnic groups, taking into account climatological and geographical conditions of residence. We studied the concentration of gonadotropins - follicle stimulating hormone (FSH), luteinising hormone (LH), prolactin, estradiol, progesterone, 17-OH-progesterone (17-OP); thyroid hormones - thyrotropic hormone

(TTH), total triiodothyronine (T3), total thyroxine (T4); androgens - testosterone, dihydroepiandrosterone (DHEA-C); steroid hormone - cortisol.

Women were examined in accordance with the recommendations for laboratory tor testing of female sex hormones on an empty stomach, between 8 and 10 am. Venous blood sampling was performed in the procedure room in the volume of 10 ml in three brief but every 30 minutes. In order to exclude variability of the data, the examination was carried out on the 3-5th days of the menstrual cycle: luteinising hormone (LH), follicle-stimulating hormone (FSH), estradiol, prolactin, testosterone and on the 20-22nd day of the cycle progesterone. Once serum samples were obtained, they were stored at -20° C.

Hormone levels were determined ***by solid-phase immunoassay*** using immobilised monoclonal antibodies and other reagents produced by DRG and a set of equipment (tablet photometer "OPSYS MR" (reader) manufactured by "THERMOLABSYSTEMS", tablet vosher PP2-428 manufactured by "IMMEDTECH", printer "EPSON") in accordance with the instructions for use of devices and reagents. The results were processed automatically using the DRGELIZAMAT instrument with its computer software DRGRegressionProgram.

Determination of follicle stimulating hormone (FSH). Monoclonal antibodies specific to the unique antigenic determinant of the β-subunit of FSH are immobilised on the surface of the wells of a microtitre plate, which acts as a solid phase. When serum samples containing endogenous FSH and an enzyme conjugate (polyclonal antibodies to FSH labelled with horseradish peroxidase) were added to the wells, the incubation resulted in the formation of a sandwich-type triple immune complex immobilised on the solid phase. After removal of unbound material by washing, the amount of bound conjugate (proportional to the concentration of FSH in the sample) is determined by adding a peroxidase substrate (tetramethylbenzidine), which initiates the reaction to form a blue-coloured reaction product. The intensity of the staining is directly proportional to the concentration of FSH in the sample ces. The enzymatic reaction is stopped by adding 50 μl of stop solution to each well.

The optical density is read at a wavelength of 450±10 nm on a microplate reader within 10 minutes of stopping the reaction. The results are processed and calculated by plotting a standard curve with the mean absorbance from each reference standard against its concentration in ng/ml with absorbance value and concentration. The concentration of FSH is quantified in mIU/ml relative to a number of reference standards.

Determination of luteinising hormone (LH). Monoclonal antibodies specific to the unique antigenic determinant of the β-subunit of LH are immobilised on the surface of the wells of a micro rotiter plate, which act as a solid phase. When serum samples containing endogenous LH and an enzyme conjugate (polyclonal antibodies to LH labelled with horseradish peroxidase) were added to the wells, incubation resulted in the formation of a sandwich-type triple immune complex immobilised on the solid phase. After removal of unbound material by washing, the amount of bound gate (proportional to the concentration of LH in the sample) is determined by adding le peroxidase substrate (tetramethylbenzidine), which initiates the reaction formation of a blue-coloured reaction product. The enzyme reaction is stopped by adding 50 μl of stop solution to each well at the same time intervals.

Optical density was read at a wavelength of 450±10 nm on a micro plan shet reader within 10 minutes after stopping the reaction. The results were processed and counted in an automated way. The intensity of staining is directly proportional to the concentration of LH in the sample. This concentration is quantified in mIU/ml relative to a number of reference standards.

Determination of the lactogenic hormone prolactin. Monoclonal antibodies specific to the unique antigenic site of the prolactin molecule are immobilised li zo on the surface of the wells of the microtitre plate, which act as a solid phase. When serum samples containing endogenous prolactin and an enzyme conjugate (polyclonal antibodies to prolactin labelled with horseradish peroxidase) are added to the wells, incubation results in the formation of a sandwich-type triple immune complex immobilised on the solid phase. After removal of unbound material by washing, the amount of bound conjugate (proportional to the concentration of prolactin in the sample) is determined by adding peroxidase substrate, which initiates the reaction to form a blue coloured reaction product.

Optical density is read at a wavelength of 450±10 on a microplate reader within 10 minutes after the reaction has stopped. The results are processed and calculated by plotting a standard curve plotting the average absorbance from each reference standard against its concentration in ng/ml with the absorbance value and concentration.

Estradiol definition. A search amount of estradiol in blood and its fixed amount in estradiol conjugate with horseradish peroxidase compete for the active centres of polyclonal anti-estradiol serum, which is sorbed on micropanels. After 2 hours of incubation, washing is performed to stop the competition reaction. After addition of the enzyme-substrate solution, the concentration of estradiol is determined as a value inversely proportional to the intensity of the resulting optical density staining. The reaction is stopped by adding 50 μl of the residual solution to each well at equal time intervals and measuring the optical density (OD) in the wells at a wavelength of 450 ± 10nm. The OD measurements shall be carried out not later than 10 minutes after completion of work with the stopping solution. The results are processed automatically using the DRGELIZAMAT instrument with its computer software DRGRegressionProgram.

Progesterone definition. A search amount of progesterone in blood and its fixed amount in the conjugate of progesterone with horseradish peroxidase compete for the active centres of polyclonal anti-progesterone serum, which is sorbed on micropanels. After 2 hours of incubation, washing is performed to stop the competition reaction. After addition of the enzyme-substrate solution, the concentration of progesterone is determined as a value inversely proportional to the intensity of the resulting staining by optical density at a wavelength of 450±10nm. OD measurements are carried out not later than 10 minutes after completion of work with stopping solution. The results are processed automatically using the DRGELIZAMAT instrument with its computer software DRGRegressionProgram.

Testosterone determination. The determination of free testosterone is based wa but on the use of a competitive enzyme immunoassay. Mouse monoclonal anti- antibodies to testosterone are immobilised on the inner surface of the wells of the plate. Free testosterone from the sample competes with conjugated gi bound testosterone for binding to the antibodies. This results in the formation of a plastic-bound "sandwich" containing peroxidase. During incubation with tetramethylbenzidine (TMB) solution, staining of the solutions in the wells occurs. The intensity of staining is inversely proportional to the concentration of free testosterone in the test sample. The OD of the contents of the wells of the plate wells is measured within 15 min after application of the stop reagent on a vertical scanning photometer at a wavelength of 450 nm. The concentration of free testosterone in the test samples is determined by the calibration graph of the dependence of optical density on the content of free testosterone in the calibration samples.

Determination of dihydroepiandrosterone sulphate (DHEA-C). The principle of the method is based on the competition of DGEA-C from the measured sample and peroxidase-labelled DGEA-C for the binding centres of antibodies specific to dehydroepiandrosterone sulphate immobilised on the surface of the wells of a polystyrene well plate. The amount of bound conjugate is detected using the substrate 3,3`,5,5`-tetramethylbenzidine (TMB). The colour intensity of the products of the enzymatic reaction of substrate oxidation is inversely proportional to the concentration of dehydroepiandrosterone sulphate contained in the sample being analysed. The OD of the plate wells is measured within 15 min after the stop reagent is applied on a vertical scanning photometer at a wavelength of 450 nm. The concentration of free testosterone in the test samples is determined by the calibration graph of the dependence of optical density on the content of free testosterone in the calibration samples.

Determination of thyroid hormone (TSH). **The** reagents required for the immunoassay include highly purified and specific anti-bodies in excess (enzyme-conjugated and immobilised) to recognise different individual epitopes and natural antigen. During the assay, immobilisation occurs on the surface of the microcells by interaction between streptavidin, which coats the cells, and the added exogenous biotinylated anti-TTG antibodies. When monoclonal biotinylated ni lated antibodies, an enzyme conjugate and serum containing the native venous antigen are mixed, a reaction (without competition or spatial difficulties) occurs between the native antigen and antibodies to form a solute ri mo sandwich complex. The interaction is illustrated by the following equation: ka EnzAb(p)+AgTSH+BtnAb(m) EnzAb(p) - AgTSH - BtnAb(m) k-a where BtnAb(m) = biotinylated monoclonal antibody (excess amount); AgTSH = native antigen (variable amount); EnzAb(p) = enzyme-labelled polyclonal antibody (excess amount); EnzAb(p) -AgTSH - BtnAb(m) = sandwich antigen-antibody complex;

ka = association rate constant cyation; k -a = dissociation rate constant. At the same time, the complex is reversed in cells due to the high affinity reaction of streptavidin and biotinylated antibodies.

This interaction is illustrated by the equation: EnzAb(p) - AgTSHBtnAb(m) + StreptavidinC.W. ⇒ immobilised complex where StreptavidinC.W. = streptavidin immobilised on cells Immobilized complex = sandwich complex bound to a solid surface. After equilibrium is reached, the antibody-bound fraction is separated from unbound antigens by decantation or washing. The enzyme activity in the bound antibody fraction is directly proportional to the native antigen concentration. The absorbance of the cell contents is measured at 450 nm (reference wavelength 620-630 nm). Measurements should be performed within 30 minutes after addition of the stop solution.

Determination of total triiodothyronine (T3). A competitive ELISA using immobilised T3 antibodies, T3 enzyme conjugate and native T3 antigen is used. When immobilised antibodies, enzyme T3-conjugate and serum containing free T3 antigen are mixed, a competitive reaction occurs between the native free T3 antigen and the enzyme conjugate for a limited number of binding sites.

The interaction is illustrated by the following equation: ka EnzAg + Ag + AbC.W. AgAbC.W. + EnzAgAbC.W AgAbC.W. k-a Abc.w - monospecific immobilised antibodies (constant amount) Ag - native free antigen (variable amount) EnzAg - antigen-enzyme conjugate (constant amount) AgAbc.w. - antigen-antibody complex EnzAgAbc.w. - comp lex antigen-enzyme conjugate - antibody Ka - association rate constant K-a - dissociation rate constant K = Ka / K-a = equilibrium constant After equilibrium is reached, the bound antibody fraction is separated from unbound antigens by decantation or aspiration. The enzyme activity in the bound antibody fraction is inversely proportional to the native free antigen concentration.

The absorbance of the cell contents is measured within 30 minutes after addition of the stop solution at a wavelength of 450 nm When using several standards with a known value of antigen concentration, a calibration curve is constructed, from which the concentration of unknown samples is calculated.

Determination of total thyroxine (T4). Principle of the method: when immobilised antibodies, enzyme conjugate and serum containing native free antigen are mixed, a competitive reaction for immobilised antibody binding sites occurs between native free antigen and enzyme-antigen conjugate . The interaction is illustrated by the following equation: ka EnzAg + Ag + AbC.W. AgAbC.W. + EnzAgAbC.W. k-a AbC.W. = monospecific immobilised antibody (constant amount) Ag = native antigen (variable amount) EnzAg = enzyme-antigen conjugate (constant amount) AgAbC.W. = antigen-antibody complex EnzAg AbC.W. = enzyme-antigen-antigen-antibody conjugate complex ka = association rate constant k-a = dissociation rate constant K = ka / k-a = equilibrium constant Once equilibrium is reached, the antibody-bound fraction is separated from the unbound antigen by decantation or washing. The enzyme activity in the antibody-bound fraction is inversely proportional to the concentration of native antigen. If several standards with known antigen concentrations are used, a calibration curve is constructed from which the concentration of the samples to be tested is calculated.

Determination of the steroid hormone cortisol. The determination method is based on solid-phase competitive enzyme immunoassay using monoclonal antibodies. In the wells of the plate, upon addition of the test sample and conjugate, competitive binding of serum cortisol and peroxidase-conjugated cortisol with monoclonal antibodies to cortisol immobilised on the inner surface of the wells occurs. During incubation with tetramethylbenzidine solution, staining of the solution in the wells occurs. The degree of staining is inversely proportional to the concentration of cortisol in the analysed samples. Measure the value of optical density of solutions in wells of strips on a vertical scanning spectrophotometer at a wavelength of 450 nm. The measurement is carried out 2 - 3 min after stopping the reaction. After measuring the optical density of the solution in the wells, the concentration of cortisol in the analysed samples is calculated on the basis of the calibration graph.

2.3.3 Methods for assessing immune status

Venous blood was subjected to the study. Blood preparation for the study was carried out by hardware method using BD FACS Sample Prep Assistant II automatic sample preparation station (Becton Dickinson, USA).

The phenotypic composition of lymphocytes was studied using zo ***flow cytofluorimeter*** BD FACSCanto II (Becton Dickinson, USA). Determination was carried out on the basis of a standardised set of mono clo antibodies (MCAT) BD Multitest 6-Color TBNK Reagent (BD Bioscien ces), which allowed to simultaneously determine the content of CD45+CD3+, CD45+CD3+CD4+, CD45+CD3+CD8+, CD45+CD3+CD56+, CD45+ CD16+ CD56+, CD45+CD19+ lymphocytes in blood. Blood B1-lymphocyte counts were determined in a separate blood sample; in each case, a set of two monoclonal antibodies was used: labelled PE-Su5 anti-CD19 ICAT (IOTest, Beckman Coulter, USA) and labelled PE anti-CD5 ICAT (IOTest, Beckman Coulter, USA). The study was performed in full compliance with the instructions for use of the instruments and monoclonal antibodies.

The flow cytometry method is based on optical and fluorescence measurement of various blood cells, which cross monochromatic laser light rays in the following order together with the flow of the reaction fluid. In this case, the physical properties of all cells, their dimensionality, cytoplasmic granularity are measured on a single cell not to be stained. Blood cells are examined with a set of fluoro chromium conjugated antibodies that are directed to intra cellular and membrane components of the cells. A monodisperse suspension with cells stained with fluorescent markers was placed in a special container of a flow cytometer, from which the sample was fed through a specially designed tip under a certain pressure into the centre of the fluid flow, which moved in the same direction at high speed. Cells that were picked up by the flow of special liquid formed a chain, and each cell formed a liquid "shell". The processed data were automatically recorded, analysed and presented in the form of special one-dimensional histograms where the abscissa axis shows the fluorescence intensity of haematological cells and the ordinate axis shows the number of haematological cells with a certain fluorescence intensity as

Immunoglobulin levels of IgM, IgG, IgA classes were studied ***by solid-phase immunoenzyme analysis*** using sets of immobilised monoclonal antibodies and other reagents produced by VectorBest (Russia) and a set of equipment (tablet OPSYS MR photometer (reader) manufactured by THERMOLABSYSTEMS, tablet tablet PP2-428 vosher manufactured by "IMMEDTECH", printer "EPSON") in accordance with the instructions for use of instruments and reagents.

In the first step, calibration samples with known concentrations of IgA, IgG, IgM and the samples to be analysed are incubated in wells of a stripped plate with immobilised monoclonal antibodies (MCAT) to IgA, IgG, IgM. The tablet is then washed. In the second step, IgA, IgG, IgM bound in the wells are treated with peroxidase conjugate of MCATs to the light (lambda and kappa) chains of human immunoglobulins. After washing off the excess conjugate, the formed immune complexes "immobilised ICAT- IgA, IgG, IgM - conjugate" are detected by enzymatic reaction of peroxidase with hydrogen peroxide in the presence of chromogen (tetramethylbenzidine). The colour intensity of the chromogen is proportional to the concentration of IgA, IgG, IgM in the analysed sample . After stopping the peroxidase reaction with a stop reagent, the results are taken into account spectrometrically. The concentration of IgA, IgG, IgM in the samples is determined according to the calibration graph.

2.3.4 Methods for assessing autoantibody levels and other markers of antiphospholipid reactions

In assessing the role of autoimmune component in reproductive health disorders, we studied the levels of autoantibodies to thyroglobulin, thyroperoxidase, as well as the total concentration of IgG class antiphospholipid antibodies to cardio lipin, phosphatidylserine, phosphatidylinositol and phosphatidiol acid, antibodies to cofactors: β-2-glycoprotein-I and annexin-V, prothrombin. Paral lel but determination of lupus-type anticoagulants in plasma was performed.

Determination of autoantibody levels to various components of own biological fluids and tissues was carried out by ***indirect immunoenzyme analysis*** using the principle of indirect solid phase ELISA-ELISA on BioRad analyser, manufactured by SanofiDiagnosticsPasteur (France - USA) using a set of reagents and monoclonal firm "Orgentec" in accordance with the instructions for use of devices and reagents.

Determination of autoantibody levels to thyroid components - thyroglobulin and thyroperoxidase. The method is based on the principle of indirect two-stage enzyme immunoassay. Specific antibodies to thyroglobulin in the serum sample or calibrator under study bind to purified thyroglobulin immobilised on the surface of microplate wells. Unbound serum proteins are removed by washing. A conjugate of horseradish peroxidase-labelled goat antibody to human IgG is then added to the wells and binds to the antigen-antibody complex immobilised on the well surface. The unbound conjugate is removed by washing.

The addition of substrate results in a colour whose intensity is directly proportional to the concentration of specific antibodies to thyroglobulin or thyroperoxidase. The concentration of antibodies to thyroglobulin or thyroo peroxidase in the samples tested is calculated from the calibration curve.

Determination of IgG class total autoantibodies to cardiolipin, phosphatidylserine, phosphatidylinositol, and phosphatidylic acid. We used plates whose cells were coated with highly purified human ve phospholipids (cardiolipin, phosphatidylserine, phosphati dily nositol and phosphatidylic acid). Antibodies to phospholipids require β2-glycoprotein-I as a cofactor, so cells were saturated with highly purified human β-2-glycoprotein-I. The plate was divided into 12 strips of 8 cells each. Binding of autoantibodies present in the assay was performed.

Sandwich complex formation and enzyme colour reaction occurred in the following reaction phases.

Phase 1- Calibrators, controls and pre-diluted patient serum samples were introduced into microcells. Any antibodies present were bound to the antigens immobilised in the microcells. After a 30-minute incubation, the cells were washed, with the washing solution removing unbound serum components.

Phase 2: A solution of anti-human-IgG conjugate with peroxidase was added to the cells for the detection of autoantibodies associated with immobilised called antigens. After a 15-minute incubation, excess enzyme conjugate was removed with washing solution.

Phase 3: The chromogenic substrate solution containing TMB was added to the cells. During the 15 min incubation, the colour of the solution turned blue. The colour development was stopped by adding

1M hydrochloric acid as a stop solution and incubated for 15 minutes. The solution changed colour to yellow. The colour intensity was directly proportional to the concentration of IgG antibodies in the sample and the optical density was determined at 450 nm wavelength of the spectrometer and the results were calculated.

Determination of class IgG autoantibodies to β2-glycoprotein I. **The** method was developed for semi-quantitative determination of total class G autoantibodies to β2-glycoprotein I. The cells of the tablet were coated with highly purified β-2 -glycoprotein I. The tablet is used for 96 determinations at once. The assay binds the autoantibodies present.

Sandwich complex formation and enzyme colour reaction in the following reaction phases: Phase 1 - Controls and pre-diluted patient serum samples were introduced into microcells. Any antibodies present were bound to the antigens immobilised in the microcells. After a 30-minute incubation, the cells were washed. The washing solution removed unbound serum components. Phase 2: a mixed solution of anti-human-IgG conjugate with peroxidase was added to the cells to determine fission of autoantibodies bound to immobilised antigens. After a 15-minute incubation, excess enzyme conjugate was removed with washing solution. Phase 3: chromogenic substrate solution containing TMB was added to the cells. During the 15 minute incubation, the colour of the solution turned blue. The colour development was stopped by adding 1M hydrochloric acid as a stop solution. The solution changed colour to yellow. The intensity of the colouring, determined by spectrophotometer at a wavelength of 450 nm, is directly proportional to the concentration of IgG antibodies present in the sample.

Determination of class IgG autoantibodies to annexin V. **The** assay binds autoantibodies present in the blood to highly purified human recombinant annexin V, which coats the cells of the plate.

The reaction proceeds in three phases.

Phase 1 - Calibrators, controls and pre-diluted patient serum samples are introduced into microcells. The antibodies present bind to the antigens immobilised in the microcells. After 30 minutes incubation, the cells are washed. The washing solution removes the unbound components of the serum.

Phase 2: A solution of anti-human-IgG conjugate with peroxidase is added to the cells for the determination of autoantibodies bound to immobilised antigens. After 15 minutes incubation, excess enzyme conjugate is removed with washing solution.

Phase 3: The chromogenic substrate solution containing TMB was added to the cells. During the 15 min incubation, the colour of the solution turned blue. The colour development was stopped by adding 1M hydrochloric acid as a stop solution. The solution changed colour to yellow. The colour intensity, directly proportional to the concentration of IgG antibodies in the sample, is determined spectro metrically at a wavelength of 450 nm.

Determination of class IgG autoantibodies to prothrombin. Tablet cells coated with highly purified human recombinant prothrombin are used. The assay involves binding of the autoantibodies present and formation of a sandwich complex followed by enzymatic colour reaction in the following phases.

Phase 1 - Calibrators, controls and pre-diluted patient serum samples are introduced into microcells to bind serum autoantibodies to the antigens immobilised in the microcells. After 30 minutes incubation, the cells are washed. The washing solution removes unbound serum components.

Phase 2: a solution of anti-human-IgG conjugate with peroxidase is added to the cells to detect autoantibodies bound to immobilised anti-genes. After a 15-minute incubation, excess enzyme conjugate is removed with washing solution.

Phase 3: The chromogenic substrate solution containing TMB was added to the cells. During the 15 min incubation, the colour of the solution turned blue. The colour development is stopped by adding 1M hydrochloric acid as a stop solution. The solution changes colour to yellow. The intensity of the colouration is directly proportional to the concentration of IgG antibodies in the sample when the wells are examined using a spectrophotometer at a wavelength of 450 nm. The results are then calculated.

For screening of lupus-type anticoagulants, the Express-Lupus test™ and prothrombin test with diluted viper venom (lebetox test) were used.

The determination of ***lupus*** anticoagulant in the original screening gov variant (***Express-Lupus-test***™) is based on a comparative evaluation of the results of registration of activated partial thromboplastin time (APTV) in the plasma of the tested person with two reagents: highly sensitive to lupus anticoagulant (APTVVA+) and low-sensitive to it (APTVVA-).

The presence of HA in plasma leads to a relatively longer clotting time in the test with APTVBA+ than with APTVBA-reagent. The difference in the clotting time obtained when performing APTV with different APTV reagents (sensitive to the action of VA and low sensitive to the action of VA) makes it possible to calculate the NR index [10]. which in our studies at values of 1.5 U indicates the presence of lupus anticoagulant in the tested plasma.

The progress of the work involves several stages:

Step 1: 0.1 ml of patient plasma is introduced into the coagulometer cuvette; incubated at +37° C for 1 min; 0.1 ml of $APTV_{BA+}$ - room temperature reagent is added; incubated at +37° C for 3 min.0.1 ml of working solution of calcium chloride (preliminarily heated to +37 ° C) is added to the mixture and the clotting time is recorded; similarly (using $APTV_{BA+}$ -reagent) the clotting time is determined in control normal plasma (or RNP-plasma).

Step 2: 0.1 ml of patient plasma is added to the coagulometer cuvette; incubated at +37° C for 1 min.Add 0.1 ml of diluted $APTV_{BA-}$ -reagent having room temperature; incubate at +37° C for 3 min; add 0.1 ml of working solution of calcium chloride (having temperature +37° C) to the mixture and record the clotting time; similarly (using $APTV_{BA-}$ -reagent) determine the clotting time in control normal plasma (or RNP-plasma of LLC firm "Technologiya-Standart", cat. no. 012). № 012).

The *NR* indicator is calculated according to the formulas:

$$R_1 = \frac{t_1}{t_2}; \quad R_2 = \frac{t_3}{t_4}; \quad NR = \frac{R_1}{R_2},$$

where: t_1 - clotting time of patient plasma with APTV reagent_{BA+} ;

t_2 - clotting time of control normal plasma with APTV reagent_{BA+}

;

t_3 - clotting time of patient plasma with APTV reagent_{BA-} ;

t_4 - clotting time of control normal plasma with APTV reagent_{BA-}

;

R_1 is the index of prolongation of clotting time in the patient, compared to the control, in the test with APTV -reagent; $_{BA+}$

R_2 . index of clotting time prolongation in the patient, compared with the control, in the test with APTV -reagent; $_{BA-}$

NR is a ratio that quantifies the hypocoagulation effect of VA.

The principle of the ***lebetox test*** is to determine the clotting time of platelet-rich recalcified citrate plasma under the influence of a solution of gyurza venom (lebetox). To obtain platelet-rich plasma, venous blood is drawn into a tube containing 3.8% sodium citrate in a blood to sodium citrate volume ratio of 9:1.

The blood is centrifuged at 1000 rpm (240 g) for 7 min to obtain platelet-rich plasma. A prolongation of the lebetox time may be due, in particular, to the presence of a lupus-type anticoagulant in the blood. In parallel, lebetox time is determined in control normal plasma [10]. In our studies, the lebetox time of coagulation in manual examination should not exceed 3 minutes.

The course of the determination includes the following procedures. 0.1 ml of lebetox solution is added to 0.1 ml of tested plasma taken into a test tube. The tube is shaken and placed for 30 seconds in a water bath at a temperature of +37° C. 0.1 ml of 0.277% calcium chloride solution (pre-warmed in a water bath at +37° C) is added to the mixture and a stopwatch is started. Note the time of coagulation (fibrin formation) with periodic shaking of the test tube. In parallel, determine the lebetox time in control normal plasma. Slowdown of clotting in comparison with the control by more than 1.2 times can be associated with the action of lupus anticoagulant.

2.4 Mathematical and statistical processing data analysis

When comparing indicators with different units of measurement, the percentage of deviation of indicators in risk groups from the control (PO, taken as 100%) was calculated according to formula 1:

Formula 1

$$ПО = \frac{\text{Показатель в группе риска} - \text{Показатель в группе контроля}}{\text{Показатель в группе контроля}} x100\%+100\%$$

Statistical processing of the data was carried out using the statistical package ti SPSS (version 21) in accordance with the instructions for its use me .

When determining the range of reference values, an interactive analysis of the entire set of obtained **OLAP-cube** data was used.

To determine the degree of informativeness of the studied factors and quantitative honest venous indices, analysis of variance with calculation of the standardised canonical coefficient of discriminant function (SCCDF) was performed.

In order to form study groups according to the analysed data, cluster analysis was used, taking into account the most informative indicators.

For statistical processing of quantitative data we used the methods of discriminative statistics with the definition of median, minimum and maximum indicators.

Comparison of values due to the absence of normal distribution of data was performed using nonparametric statistics. When analysing the frequencies of data, a one-factor analysis of variance (ONE WAY ANOVA) was used to determine the homogeneity or heterogeneity of the distribution of the frequency of occurrence of a feature in the compared groups using the Fisher criterion. The Mann-Whitney test was used to analyse quantitative indicators. Differences were considered reliable at $p < 0.05$.

To develop a methodology for calculating integral markers of reproductive health disorders, regression analysis was used to obtain a linear regression equation within each population and the corresponding risk groups.

To determine the prognostically significant range of laboratory values and markers, their 95% confidence interval was calculated.

The ratio of sensitivity and specificity of the obtained criteria in assessing the prognostic accuracy of each informative sign or indicator was established by linear regression method with ROC-curve construction and calculation of the area under the curve - AUROC [80, 219, 342].

CHAPTER 3. PRENOSOLOGICAL AND POPULATION-CLUSTER APPROACH TO ASSESSING WOMEN'S REPRODUCTIVE HEALTH

3.1. Methodological bases of prenosological assessment Reproductive health of women in different populations

Since the aim of the study was to investigate the reproductive health of women at the prenosological stage, first of all, an attempt was made to clarify the physiological norms (reference values) of the studied indicators for women of fertile age belonging to the Russian and Tajik populations.

For this purpose, interactive data analysis (On-Line Analytical Processing - **OLAP-cube**) was used, according to which the interval of reference values was in the range X±σ (mean ± standard deviation).

In accordance with this information, data from 510 clinically healthy women living in the Middle Black Earth Region of Russia (Russian population) and 515 healthy women living in Tajikistan (Tajik population) were analysed.

Hormonal status was firstly determined in all these women within each population, and on the basis of the data obtained, a range of reference values was formed for each population under study, as presented in Table 1. Figures 1 and 2 show the percentages of deviation of the obtained reference ranges of hormonal status indicators for each bullet from the reference ranges of the same indicators recommended in current literature sources.

As follows from the table and figure, in general, the range of variation in the reference values of the indicators in our studies was somewhat narrower than indicated in the literature, which is quite understandable due to the limitations of the population of women.

Table 1. Reference ranges of blood hormonal status indicators in women of different populations

Tested laboratory value	Reference values recommended in the literature	Refined reference values	
		X ± σ	Established population range
Population of Russian women			
Follicle-stimulating hormone (FSH), IU/L	3,5 - 6,0	4,8 ± 1,7	3,1 - 6,1
Luteinising hormone (LH), IU/L	4,0 - 9,0	4,8 ± 1,4	3,4 - 6,2
Prolactin, nmol/l	120 - 500	208,9 ± 107,4	101,5 - [illegible]
Estradiol, pmol/l	228 - 400	268,6 ± 46,0	222.6 - 314,6
Progesterone, nmol/l	20 - 90	37,4 ± 18,9	18,5 - 56,3
17-OH-progesterone (17-OP), nmol/L	2,0-3,3	2,8 ± 1,3	1,5 - 4,1
Testosterone, nmol/l	1,5 - 2,5	2,1 ± 1,3	0,8 - 3,4
Dihydroepiandrosterone (DHEA-C), nmol/L	1,3 - 6,0	4,5 ± 1,8	2,7 - 6,3
Thyroid hormone (TSH), mIU/L	0,4 - 4,0	1,8 ± 1,77	0,03 - 3,57
Total triiodothyronine (total T3), nmol/l	2,0 - 3,3	2,0 ± 1,3	0,7 - 3,3
Total thyroxine (total T4), nmol/L	77 - 142	101,9 ± 24,2	77,7 - 126,1
Cortisol, nmol/l	200 - 400	272,0 ± [illegible]	208,4 - [illegible]
Population of Tajik women			
Follicle-stimulating hormone (FSH), IU/L	3,5 - 6,0	3,9 ± 1,6	2,3 - 5,5
Luteinising hormone (LH), IU/L	4,0 - 9,0	5,0 ± 1,4	3,6 - 6,4
Prolactin, nmol/l	120 - 500	172,6 ± 51,6	121,0 - 224,2
Estradiol, pmol/l	228 - 400	240,8 ±	228,0 -
Progesterone, nmol/l	20 - 90	29,2 ± 8,8	20,4 - 38,0
17-OH-progesterone (17-OP), nmol/L	2,0-3,3	3,1 ± 1,0	2,0 - 4,6
Testosterone, nmol/l	1,5 - 2,5	2,3 ± 1,0	1,3 - 3,3
Dihydroepiandrosterone (DHEA-C), nmol/L	1,3 - 6,0	4,9 ± 1,9	3,0 - 6,8
Thyroid hormone (TSH), mIU/L	0,4 - 4,0	1,6 ± 1,3	0,3 - 2,9
Total triiodothyronine (total T3), nmol/l	2,0 - 3,3	2,3 ± 1,0	1,3 - 3,3
Total thyroxine (total T4), nmol/L	77 - 142	104,4 ± 25,5	78,8 - 120,0

Cortisol, nmol/l	200 - 400	278,0 ± 63,9	214,3 - 341,9

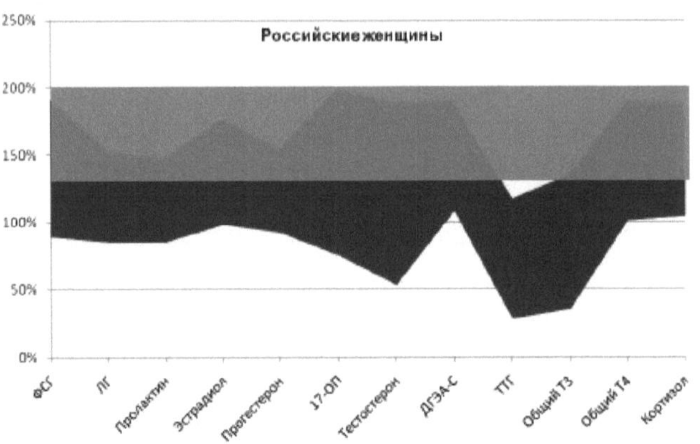

Fig. 1. Reference values of hormonal status indicators in women of the Russian population (blue colour) in comparison with literature data (green colour)

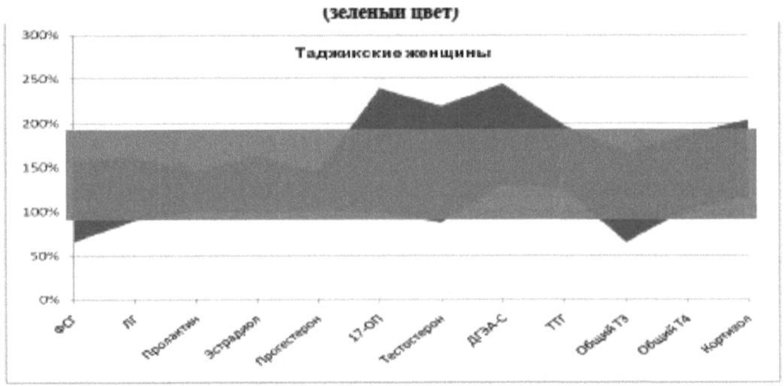

Fig. 2. Reference values of hormonal status indicators in women of Tajik population (red colour) in comparison with with literature data (green colour)

In the population of Russian women, the reflex values of indicators for blood androgens and thyroid hormones were somewhat lower than generally accepted values, while in the population of Tajik women, on the contrary, the level of androgens in blood was significantly higher, and the content of thyroid hormones, with the exception of total triiodothyronine, corresponded to generally accepted standards.

Similarly, using interactive **OLAP-cube** data analysis, ranges of reference values for immunological parameters were obtained, which are presented as absolute values in Table 2 and as percentages of deviation from standard values in Figures 3-4.

Table 2. Reference ranges of blood immune status indicators in women of different populations

Tested laboratory value	Reference values recommended in the literature	Refined reference values	
		X ± σ	Established population range
Population of Russian women			
T-lymphocytes (CD3+), %	61 - 85	69,8 ± 4,4	65,4 - 74,2
T-helpers (CD3+CD4+), %	20 - 40	35,7 ± 2,4	33,3 - 38,1
Cytotoxic T-lymphocytes	19 - 35	21,8 ± 5,0	16,8 - 26,8
ECT (CD3+CD56+), %	1 - 6	4,2 ± 2,1	2,1 - 6,3
Natural killer cells (CD16+CD56+), %	8 - 18	13,5 ± 2,9	10,6 - 18,8
B-lymphocytes (CD19+), %	7 - 17	9,5 ± 4,1	5,4 - 13,6
B1-lymphocytes (CD19+CD5+), %	0,5 - 2,1	1,3 ± 0,3	1,0 - 1,6
IgM, mg/ml	0,5 - 1,9	1,2 ± 0,5	0,7 - 1,7
IgG, mg/ml	8 - 16	11,1 ± 2,5	8,6 - 13,6
IgA, mg/ml	0,8 - 2,8	1,7 ± 0,7	1,0 - 2,4
Population of Tajik women			
T-lymphocytes (CD3+), %	61 - 85	67,7 ± 4,1	59,0 - 71,8
T-helpers (CD3+CD4+), %	20 - 40	34,8 ± 2,1	30,1 - 37,5
Cytotoxic T-lymphocytes	19 - 35	20,4 ± 2,6	17,8 - 23,6
ECT (CD3+CD56+), %	1 - 6	3,8 ± 2,8	1,0 ± 6,6

Natural killer cells (CD16+CD56+), %	8 - 18	13,0 ± 3,7	8,7 - 20,1
B-lymphocytes (CD19+), %	7 - 17	12,7 ± 5,9	6,8 - 18,6
B1-lymphocytes (CD19+CD5+), %	0,5 - 2,1	1,8 ± 0,6	1,2 - 2,4
IgM, mg/ml	0,5 - 1,9	1,2 ± 0,4	0,5 - 1,8
IgG, mg/ml	8 - 16	11,7 ± 1,8	9,9 - 15,6
IgA, mg/ml	0,8 - 2,8	1,6 ± 0,6	0,6 - 2,4

$

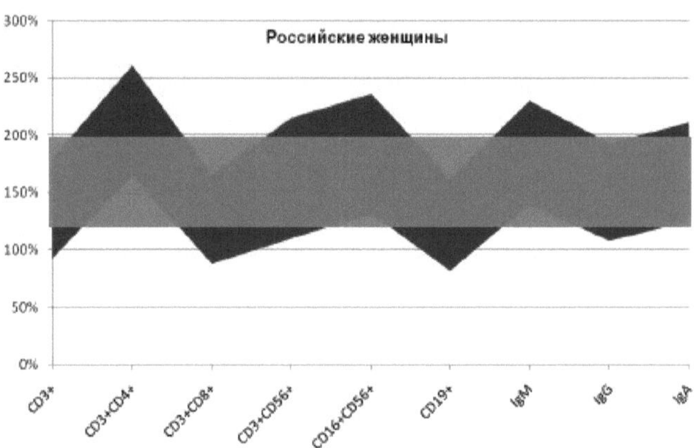

Fig. 3. Reference values of immune status indicators in women of the Russian population (blue colour) in comparison with the literature data (green colour)

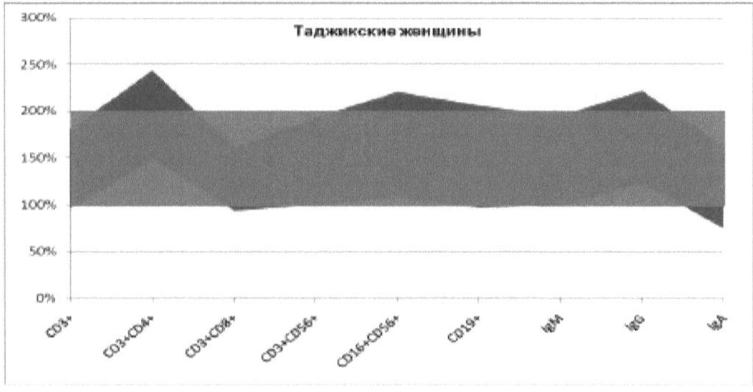

Figure 4. Reference values of immune status indicators in women of Tajik population (red colour) in comparison with with literature data (green colour)

As follows from the presented data, the deviations in the reference values of the immune status indicators obtained by us from the standard range of reference values were not very significant. In the Russian population of women, the percentage of T-helper cells, EKT, natural ven killers, and IgM levels were slightly higher, with a narrower range of variation. In the Tajik population, the most significant deviation in favour of an increase was given only by the proportion of T-helper cells in the blood.

Table 3: Reference ranges of blood autoimmune status indicators in women of different populations

Tested laboratory value	Reference values recommend ed in the literature	Refined reference values	
		X ± σ	Established population range
1	2	3	4
Population of Russian women			
IgG-autoantibodies to thyroglobulin,	≤ 4,1	4,5 ± 0,4	4,1 - 4,9
IgG autoantibodies to	≤ 18	22,2 ± 3,2	19,0 - 25,4
IgG autoantibodies to	≤ 10 units/ml	4,2 ± 2,9	1,3 - 7,1
IgG autoantibodies to	≤ 10 units/ml	4,6 ± 2,6	2,0 - 7,2
IgG autoantibodies to	≤ 5 units/ml	2,1 ± 1,1	1,0 - 3,2
IgG autoantibodies to	≤ 10 units/ml	4,3 ± 2,5	1,8 - 6,8
Lupus anitcoagulant (Lupus test)	0.7 TO 1.1 UNITS	0,95 ± 0,25	0,7 - 1,2
Lupus anitcoagulant (Lebetox test)	≤ 3 min.	1,7 ± 1,0	0,7 - 2,7
Population of Tajik women			
IgG-autoantibodies to thyroglobulin	≤ 4.1 IU/ml	3,35 ± 0,95	2,4 - 4,3
IgG autoantibodies to	≤ 18 IU/ml	16,2 ± 6,9	9,3 - 23,1
IgG autoantibodies to	≤ 10 units/ml	8,8 ± 3,1	5,7 - 11,9

IgG autoantibodies to	≤ 10 units/ml	8,85 ± 2,75	6,1 - 11,6
IgG autoantibodies to	≤ 5 units/ml	4,7 ± 1,6	3,1 - 6,3
IgG autoantibodies to	≤ 10 units/ml	8,45 ± 3,15	5,3 - 11,6
Lupus anitcoagulant (Lupus test)	0.7 TO 1.1 UNITS	1,0 ± 0,6	0,4 - 1,6
Lupus anitcoagulant (Lebetox test)	≤ 3 min.	1,9 ± 0,9	1,0 - 2,8

The last stage of this section of the research concerned the determination of the range of reference values of blood IgG autoantibodies to individual components of the thyroid gland and protein-lipid components of the haemostasis system. These data are reflected in Table 3, which shows the numerical values of the indicators, and Figures 5-6, which graphically show the percentages of deviation of the indicators of the autoimmune component of blood in the Russian and Tajik populations of women from the generally accepted standards covered in modern scientific literature.

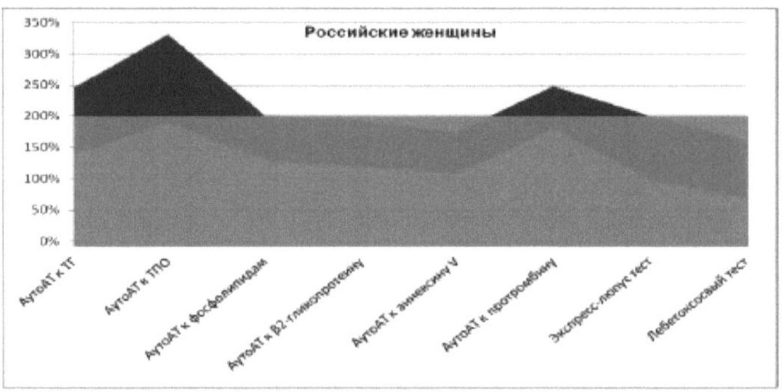

Figure 5. Reference values of autoimmune component indices in women of the Russian population (blue colour) in comparison with literature data (green colour)

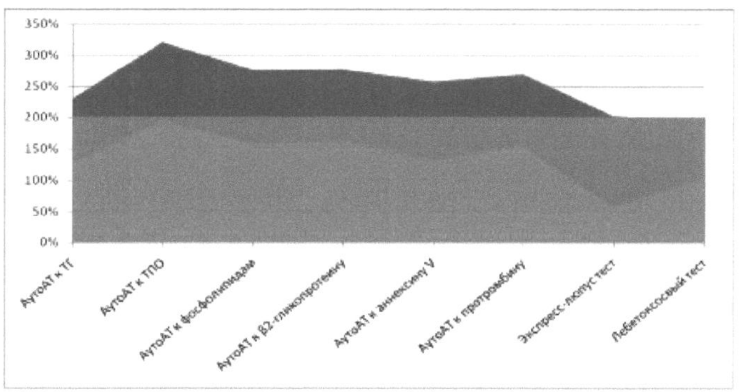

Figure 6. Reference values of autoimmune component indices in women of Tajik population (red colour) in comparison with with literature data (green colour)

As can be seen from the table and figures, the reference values of the autoimmune component in both the population of Russian women and Tajik women slightly exceeded those shown in the recommendations of other authors, with the only difference being that Russian women had higher levels of auto antibodies to thyroid components and to prothrombin, while Tajik women showed an increase in the levels of all autoantibodies tested.

Thus, these studies allowed us to clarify the reference values of hormonal status, immune status, and autoimmune component in women of the studied populations. These studies created a basis for selecting women in each population into study groups whose laboratory tor indicators were within the reference values for more than 80% of the tests, but who had differences in obstetric history.

The following groups were planned according to obstetric history in each population of women of fertile age:

1) women who gave birth and whose pregnancy/pregnancies ended in the delivery of healthy children at term - control group with preserved reproductive ive function;

2) women who have given birth and have a history of pregnancy pregnancy/ pregnancy that ended in premature labour, foetal incompletion or stillbirth - a risk group with reproductive disorders;
3) unborn women planning pregnancy and intended for observation by an obstetrician-gynaecologist during the next three years after laboratory examination - a group for testing the methods of predicting the risk of reproductive disorders proposed in this work.

It should be additionally emphasised that, despite the presence of anamnestic data on reproductive disorders in the risk group, the women in these groups had no signs of such disorders, since the results of clinical analysis and laboratory tests of their blood did not deviate significantly from the reference values, i.e. reproductive disorders, if any, were at a prenosological level. It was in these cases that the risk prediction of reproductive disorders was most needed.

The results of the selection and characterisation of the formed study groups are presented in Table 4.

Table 4: Qualitative and quantitative composition of the study groups in Russian and Tajik populations

Investigated population	Study group	Characteristics of the study group		
		Numerical compositio n	Medium age	% reference different values
Russian population	Control without	28 people.	29.3 ± 3.9 years	82,8% - 100%
	Risk group with	53 people.	29.8 ± 2.6 years	82,8% - 100%
	Monitoring the effectiveness	26 people.	22.1 ± 1.1 years	82,8% - 96,6%
Tajik population	Control without	28 people.	30.0 ± 2.7 years	82,8% - 100%

	Risk group with	57 people.	31.4 ± 5.2 years	82,8% - 96,6%
	Monitoring the effectiveness	29 people.	21.3 ± 0.9 years	82,8% - 96,6%

As shown in the table, within each population, using the inclusion/non-inclusion and exclusion criteria, it was possible to form three observation groups in which deviations from reference values were not lower than 80% of the test set.

The Russian population included 107 women out of 510, including 28 women in the control group, 53 women in the risk group, and 26 women in the prognostic performance control group. In the first 2 groups, the mean age of women was approximately equal to each other, while the group of women who did not give birth was significantly younger.

In the Tajik population, 113 women out of 515 were selected for further studies. Among them were 28 women with preserved reproductive function (control), 57 women with signs of reproductive dysfunction, and 28 unborn women to control the effectiveness of predicting the risk of reproductive disorders of approximately the same age categories as in the Russian population.

3.2 Population characteristics in women fertile

At this stage of the study, population differences in women with different ethnicity and regions of residence were determined in terms of a set of hormonal, immune traits, the presence of an autoimmune component, and immunogenetic features.

First of all, the hormonal status of women from different populations was analysed, the results of which are presented in Table 5 and Figure 7.

Table 5. Indicators of hormonal status in the blood of women belonging to different populations

Indicators hormonal status	Median indicator		p
	Russian women, n = 107	Tajik women, n = 113	
Follicle-stimulating hormone (IU/L)	4,8 [1,1; 7,7]	3,9 [0,4; 8,5]	<0,001
Luteinising hormone (IU/L)	4,5 [1,7; 8,5]	4,9 [1,4; 8,9]	0,121
Prolactin (mME/ml)	132,2 [125,8;	208,8 [121,0; 220,0]	0,146
Estradiol (pmol/l)	233,5 [200,9;	249,0 [220,3; 253,4]	0,140
Progesterone (nmol/l)	24,5 [19,1; 56,7]	34,7 [17,9; 39,3]	0,019
17-OP (nmol/l)	2,6 [0,2; 6,6]	3,1 [0,7; 5,0]	0,015
Testosterone (nmol/l)	2,0 [0,2; 6,6]	2,0 [0,1; 5,2]	0,643
DHEAc (nmol/l)	3,6 [1,7; 6,4]	4,4 [2,0; 8,9]	<0,001
Thyroid hormone (mME/l)	0,8 [0,1; 5,2]	1,3 [0,1; 3,1]	0,007
Total triiodothyronine (nmol/ml)	1,7 [0,1; 7,0]	1,9 [0,1; 3,8]	0,660
Total thyroxine (nmol/l)	85,5 [81,7; 127,2]	99,7 [78,0; 120,0]	0,102
Cortisol (nmol/l)	317,4 [207,4;	251,0 [244,1; 350,0]	0,310

Note: n - number of women in the group; p - probability of differences in the comparison groups; grey colour indicates the reliability of differences by the Mann-Whitney test at $p < 0.005$

Figure 7 shows the percentage of deviation of Russian and Tajik women's indicators from the average values.

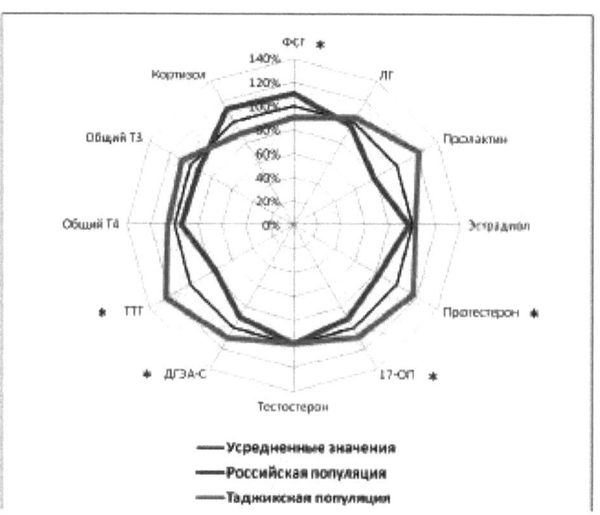

Figure 7. Percentages of deviation from the average values of indicators
Hormonal status in women of different populations
(* - differences between the values of indicators are statistically reliable)

As the data obtained showed, there were significant differences in hormonal status between the populations of Russian and Tajik women, which extended, first of all, to the level of follicle muli rulating hormone, which was significantly higher in Russian women. In addition, significant differences were noted for the levels of progesterone, 17-OH-progesterone, dihydroepiandogen sulphate, and thyroid hormone, which were higher in women of the Tajik population.

Table 6 (absolute values) and Figure 8 (percentage of deviations from the average values) present the results of analyses to identify interpopulation differences in immune status indicators in Russian and Tajik women.

Table 6: Immune status indicators in the blood of women belonging to different populations

Indicators immune status	**Median indicator [minimum, maximum]**		**p**
	Russian women, n = 107	**Tajik women, n = 113**	

T-lymphocytes (CD3+), %	70,4 [64,3; 74,5]	66,1 [55,6; 75,2]	0,156
T-helpers (CD3+CD4+), %	35,7 [31,0; [illegible]]	33,6 [29,9; [illegible]]	0,112
Cytotoxic T-lymphocytes (CD3+CD8+), %	18,7 [16,1; 28,3]	21,2 [13,2; 24,3]	< 0,001
ECT (CD3+CD56+), %	3,7 [2,1; 7,0]	1,6 [0,9; 6,0]	< 0,001
Natural killer cells (CD16+CD56+), %	12,5 [10,0; 20,4]	10,6 [3,2; 22,9]	< 0,001
B-lymphocytes (CD19+), %	7,0 [4,5; 13,6]	13,2 [7,9; 19,9]	< 0,001
IgM, mg/ml	1,2 [0,1; 2,1]	1,1 [0,1; 2,7]	0,173
IgG, mg/ml	10,3 [7,9; 13,9]	12,7 [9,9; 16,3]	< 0,001
IgA, mg/ml	1,9 [0,9; 3,5]	1,2 [0,1; 3,0]	< 0,001

Note: n - number of women in the group; p - probability of differences in the comparison groups; grey colour indicates the reliability of differences by the Mann-Whitney test at p < 0.005

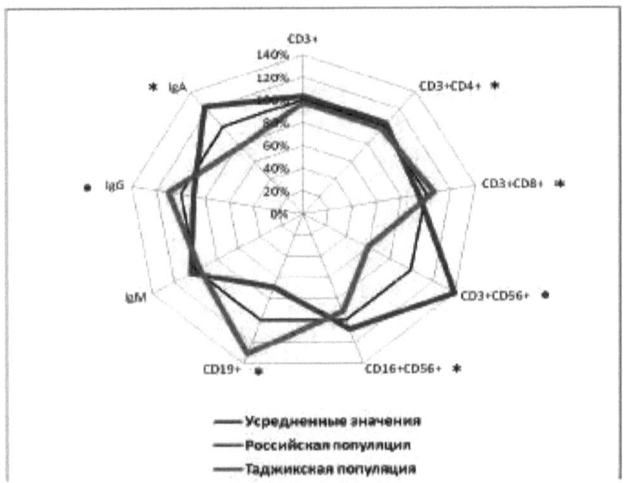

Figure 8. Percentages of deviation from the average values of indicators immune status in women of different populations
(* - differences between the values of indicators are statistically reliable)

As a result of determining possible differences between the immune status of women of different populations, it was found that the blood content of T-lymphocytes, T-helpers, and IgM levels did not differ significantly. The relative number of cytotoxic T-lymphocytes, B-cells, and IgG levels were higher in the Tajik women population, while the number of EKT and natural killer cells and IgA levels deviated quite significantly towards higher values in Russian women.

Signs of autoimmune component in the blood of women of both populations were investigated in the same way (Table 7, Figure 9).

Table 7. Autoimmune component indices in the blood of women from different populations

Indicators immune status	**Median indicator [minimum, maximum]**		**p**
	Russian women, n = 107	**Tajik women, n = 113**	
1	2	3	4
IgG-autoantibodies to thyroglobulin, IU/ml	4,6 [4,1; 5,0]	2,8 [2,6; 4,2]	< 0,001
IgG autoantibodies to thyroperoxidase, IU/ml	24,0 [10,8; 26,0]	12,3 [10,8; 41,3]	< 0,001
Total IgG autoantibodies to phospholipids	3,5 [1,0; 7,1]	7,1 [5,0; 13,8]	< 0,001
IgG autoantibodies to β_2 -glycoprotein I, units/ml	3,6 [1,2; 8,6]	7,3 [5,6; 12,6]	< 0,001
1	2	3	4
IgG autoantibodies to annexin V, units/ml	2,3 [1,0; 4,3]	4,6 [1,9; 7,5]	< 0,001
IgG autoantibodies to prothrombin, units/ml	4,2 [1,2; 8,7]	7/0 [4,7; 13,6]	< 0,001
Lupus anitcoagulant (Lupus test), units/ml	0,9 [0,6; 1,5]	1,1 [0,1; 3,9]	0,063
Lupus anitcoagulant (Lebetox test), min.	1,4 [0,4; 3,7]	1,9 [0,1; 4,2]	< 0,001

Note: n - number of women in the group; p - probability of differences in the comparison groups; grey colour indicates the reliability of differences by the Mann-Whitney test at $p < 0.005$

As can be seen from the table and figure, the reliability of differences between populations for indicators of the autoimmune component was quite pronounced and concerned almost every parameter, except for lupus anticoagulant in the express lupus test.

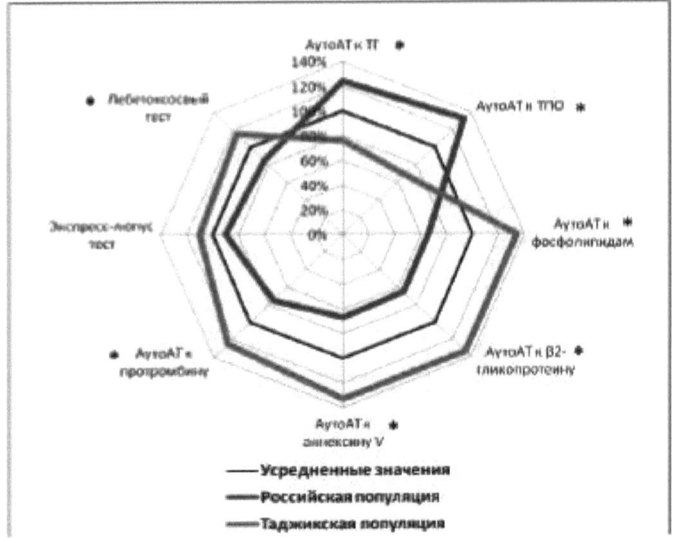

Figure 9. Percentages of deviation from the average values of indicators
autoimmune component in women of different populations
(* - differences between the values of indicators are statistically reliable)

At the same time, the level of autoantibodies to thyroid components was to correctly higher in the population of Russian women, and the levels of autoantibodies to protein kovo-lipid components of the haemostasis system, which characterise antiphospho li pid reactions, were higher in the Tajik population.

Since the main source of autoantibodies is the B_1 -subpopulation of lymphocytes [306], it would be interesting to establish how these cells are represented in the blood of women of different populations and whether differences in the variation of autoantibody levels to components of the thyroid and haemostasis system in different populations can be characterised using these quantitative measures.

The results of determining the percentage of B1-lymphocytes in the blood of women from the Russian and Tajik populations are presented in Figure 10.

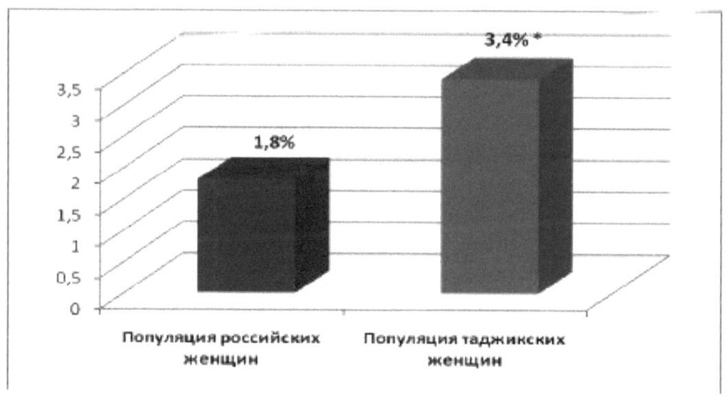

Figure 10. Content of B_1 -lymphocytes in the blood of women of different population affiliation

As follows from the figure, the content of B_1 -lymphocytes in the blood of Tajik women is almost 2 times higher than in the Russian population, which pathogenetically can be associated with a higher level of antibodies to components of haemostasis and a greater predisposition of Tajik women to the development of anti- phospholipid reaction with its ability to affect reproductive health.

A separate category of population studies was a large-scale analysis of the specific features of the studied categories of women at the genetic level. The carriage of HLA class I and II genes in women of the populations under study - 515 Russian and 510 Tajik women - was analysed.

To investigate the frequency of occurrence of genes of the major histocompatibility complex class I (MHC-I) in the populations of Russian and Tajik women, the blood of each of them was subjected to molecular genetic analysis using PCR. The results of the study comparing the carriage of these genes in representatives of different populations are reflected in Table 8.

Table 8: Frequency of occurrence of different genes of the major histocompatibility complex class I in the populations of Russian and Tajik women

Options MNS-I genes		Frequency of occurrence variants of MNS-I genes in a population of	Frequency of occurrence variants of MNS-I genes in a population of	p
1		2	3	4
HLA-A	A1	89 people / 17.3%	93 persons / 18.1	0,734
	A2	149 people / 28.6	116 people / 22.8	0,421
	A3	67 people / 13.0%	74 people / 14.5%	0,389
	A9	63 persons / 12.3%	68 people / 13.2%	0,416
	A10	83 persons / 16.2%	87 people / 17.1	0,289
	A11	14 people / 2.8 per	12 persons / 2.4%	0,754
	A19	21 persons / 4.1 per	21 persons / 4.2%	0,920
	A28	22 people / 4.3%	25 people / 4.9%	0,511
	A29	7 persons / 1.4%	14 people / 2.8 per	0,034
1		2	3	4
HLA-B	B5	37 persons / 7.1 per	36 persons / 7.1 per	0,946
	B7	20 persons / 3.9 per	17 people / 3.4%	0,564
	B8	36 people / 7.0%	37 persons / 7.3%	0,328
	B12	53 persons / 10.1 per cent	53 people / 10.2%;	0,710
	B13	28 people / 5.5%	30 persons / 5.9 per	0,345
	B14	14 persons / 2.8 per	15 persons / 2.8 per	0,879
	B15	25 people / 4.9%	27 people / 5.3%	0,253
	B16	36 people / 7.0%	42 people / 8.3%	0,212
	B17	26 people / 5.1 per	24 people / 4.7%	0.187
	B18	59 people / 11.5%	53 people / 10.2%;	0,266
	B21	15 persons, / 3.0%	16 persons / 3.2%	0.719
	B22	11 people / 2.2%	12 persons / 2.4%	0,692
	B27	37 people / 7.1 %	36 persons / 7.1 per	0,963
	B35	65 people / 12.7%	66 persons / 13.0%	0,895
	B40	53 persons / 10.1	46 persons / 9.1 per	0,289
HLA-C	Cw2	175 people / 34.0%	108 persons / 21.1	0,044
	Cw3	211 people / 41.0%	235 people / 46.1 per cent	0,217

	Cw4	12 persons / 2.4%	17 people / 3.3%	0,059
	Cw5	117 people / 22.6 per cent	150 people / 29.5 per cent	0,128

Note: n - number of women; p - probability of interpopulation differences; grey indicates the reliability of differences according to the χ^2 criterion at $p < 0.05$

As follows from the table, the differences in the frequency of occurrence of various variants of genes encoding HLA class I molecules in the populations of Russian and Tajik women were minimal. Only two significant differences were recorded: in the population of Russian women, the presence of the HLA-Cw1 gene was 1.6 times more frequent, and in the population of Tajik women, HLA-A29 was detected 2 times more frequently.

Further, allelic variants at three loci of HLA-D genes (HLA-DRB1, HLA-DQA1, HLA-DQB1) controlling the immune response were investigated. The genes associated with reproductive disorders in women - alleles HLA-DRB1*04, HLA-DQA1*103, HLA-DQA1*301, HLA-DQB1*302 - deserved special attention. The results obtained for the frequency of alleles belonging to three different loci of the HLA-D genes are shown in Figures 11-13.

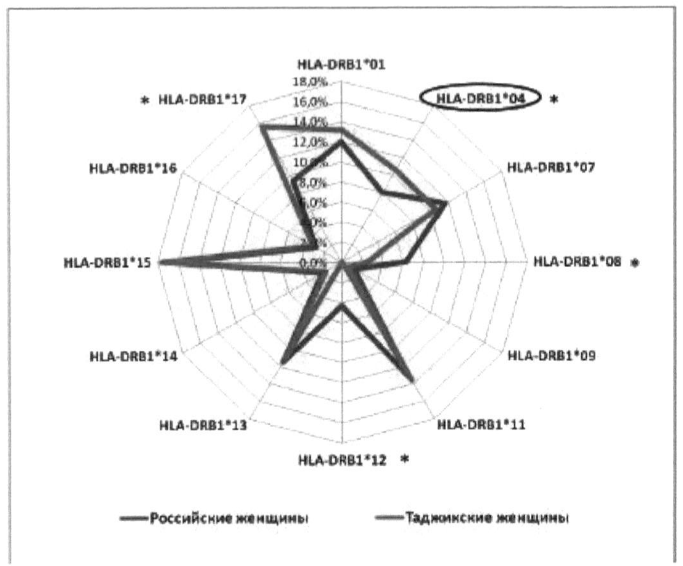

Figure 11: Frequency of occurrence of different alleles of the HLA-DRB1 locus in women of the Russian and Tajik populations

(* - differences between the values of the indicators are statistically reliable, oval alleles with unfavourable reproductive prognosis are marked)

As shown in Figure 11, there are certain population differences in the HLA-DRB1 gene locus. The HLA-DRB1*08 and HLA-DRB1*12 alleles are more frequently found in the population of Russian women, while the HLA-DRB1*17 allele was significantly more frequently registered in the population of Tajik women. .

As for the HLA-DRB1*04 allele associated with a higher incidence of non-pregnancy [11, 338], it was significantly more frequent in women of the Tajik population (1.4 times), which suggests that the genetic nature of non-pregnancy may have been slightly more frequent in the Tajik population.

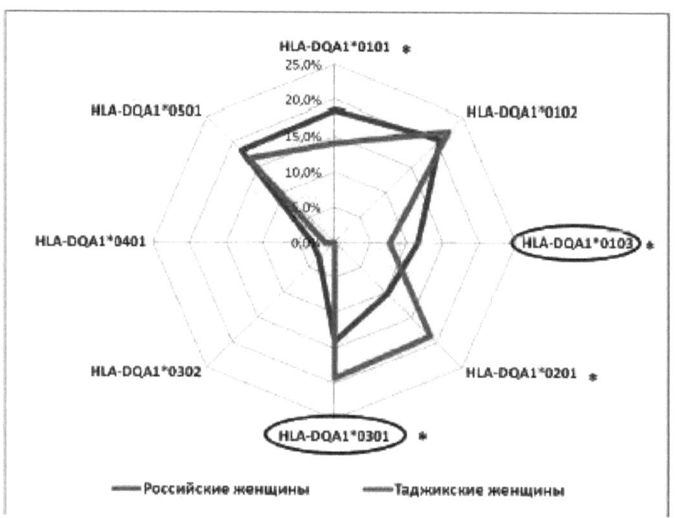

Figure 12. Frequency of occurrence of different alleles of the HLA-DQA1 locus in women of the Russian and Tajik populations
(* - differences between the values of the indicators are statistically reliable, oval
alleles with unfavourable reproductive prognosis are marked)

Figure 12 shows the presence of population peculiarities in the HLA-DQA1 gene locus. In the group of women from the Russian population, the frequency of HLA-DQA1*0101 (1.3-fold) and HLA-DQA1*0103 (1.6-fold) alleles was significantly higher, the former of which is associated with protective properties in relation to reproductive pathology, and the latter, on the contrary, with pregnancy failure. At the same time, the HLA-DQA1*0201 (1.9-fold) and HLA-DQA1*0301 (1.5-fold) alleles were significantly more frequent in the Tajik women population compared to them. As in the previous case, reproductive health disorders are not characteristic for the HLA-DQA1*0201 allele, while in the case of the HLA-DQA1*0301 allele they accompany it. In other words, variants of prevalence of undesirable alleles at this locus were registered in both Russian and Tajik populations studied.

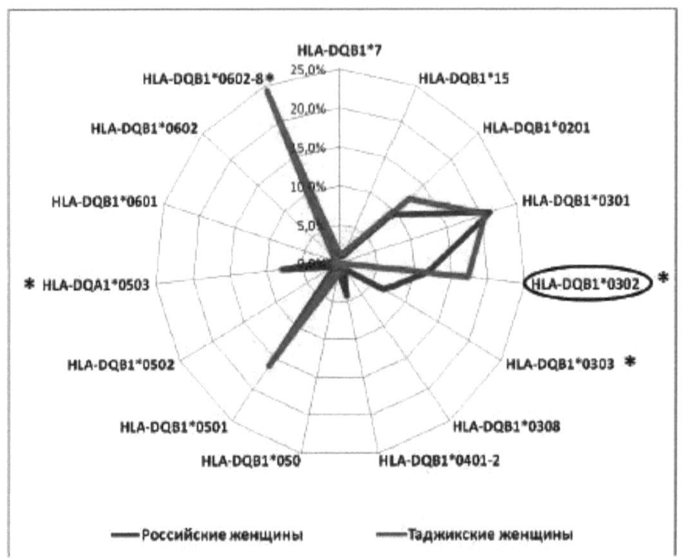

Figure 13: Frequency of occurrence of different alleles of the HLA-DQB1 locus in women of the Russian and Tajik populations

(* - differences between the values of the indicators are statistically reliable, oval alleles with unfavourable reproductive prognosis are marked)

The revealed differences between the populations at the HLA-DQB1 gene locus (Fig. 13) included a higher frequency of HLA-DQB1*0303 (7-fold) and HLA-DQB1*0503 (8-fold) alleles in Russian women, although in general it was not significant. In the population of Tajik women, alleles HLA-DQB1*0302 (1.5-fold) and HLA-DQB1*0602-8 (1.4-fold) were registered with a rather high and significantly different frequency, the former of which is considered unfavourable in association with reproductive dysfunction (non-pregnancy).

Thus, this fragment of the study allowed us to establish that there are differences between the populations of Russian and Tajik women in a number of parameters of hormonal and immune status, as well as at the level of allelic variants of genes controlling the immune response. At the same time, favourable and unfavourable alleles in terms of reproductive disorders occur with approximately equal frequency within the populations, but they were registered slightly more frequently in Tajik women.

The data obtained also show that in different populations, when assessing reproductive health, a differentiated approach is needed not only to establish physiological norms (reference values) for these categories of parameters, but also to assess women's reproductive health in general.

3.3 A cluster approach to assessing the reproductive health of women living in the Central Black Earth Region of Russia

In this section of the research, an attempt was made to develop a principle of grouping women living in the Central Black Earth Region of Russia, which would make it possible to form a risk group for threats to women's reproductive health and create, on the basis of such a forecast, the prospect of developing a system of reliable therapeutic and preventive measures.

In the population of Russian women of reproductive age, as already indicated , 107 people were monitored, of whom 28 people had all their pre six pregnancies ended in the birth of healthy children, i.e. they were women with preserved reproductive health.

Fifty-three women showed signs of reproductive health problems, as their obstetric history included either non-pregnancy, premature birth, foetal growth retardation or stillbirth.

Twenty-six women who did not give birth were also included, but this category was not included in this series of studies.

The attribute of preserved or impaired reproductive health was used as the basis for discriminant analysis of the results of the survey of 81 Russian women in the above categories. The purpose of the discriminant analysis was to identify the most informative features characterising the differences between preserved and impaired reproductive health, and the degree of discrepancy between the groups was determined according to the magnitude of the standardised canonical coefficient of discriminant function (SCCDF). Discriminant analysis allowed to reveal the signs, established new and having the greatest informativeness. The SCCDF > 0.5 was taken as a conditional value of the highest informative value .

The signs of such division by the degree of their informativeness, ranked by the value of SCCDF, are presented in Table 9, with the first 8 indicators having SCCDF values in the range above the conditional value of 0.5.

In this fragment of the study there were 8 out of 29 informative parameters for differentiation on the basis of reproductive health, and the most significant were the levels of thyroxine T4 and estradiol, as well as such immunological parameters as the content of natural killer cells and cytotoxic T-lymphocytes in the blood. This was followed by such indicators as the levels of IgG-autoantibodies to β_2 -glycoprotein 1, progesterone, autoantibodies to thyroglobulin, prolactin.

Table 9. Standardised canonical coefficients of the discriminant function of informative blood parameters in Russian women with different reproductive health statuses

Informative blood counts	[SCCDF].
1	**2**
Total thyroxine level, T4 (nmol/l)	2,602
Estradiol level (pmol/l)	2,601

Number of natural killer cells, CD16+CD56+ (%)	2,035
Number of cytotoxic T-lymphocytes, CD3+CD8+ (%)	1,471
Level of IgG autoantibodies to β_2 -glycoprotein (units/ml)	1,005
Progesterone level (nmol/l)	0,917
Thyroglobulin autoantibody level (IU/ml)	0,699
Prolactin level (mME/ml)	0,515
Number of B-lymphocytes, CD19+ (%)	0,458
Number of T-lymphocytes, CD3+ (%)	0,429
Number of ECTs, CD3+CD56+ (%)	0,419
Level of IgG-autoantibodies to thyroglobulin, IU/ml	0,352
Follicle stimulating hormone level, IU/L	0,249
IgG level, mg/ml	0,226
Luteinising hormone level, IU/L	0,210
Dihydroepiandrosterone sulphate level, nmol/L	0,209
Testosterone level, nmol/l	0,208
Lupus anticoagulant level, U/mL	0,189
17-OH progesterone level, nmol/L	0,184
Blood clotting time in lebetox test, min.	0,159
Level of IgG-autoantibodies to prothrombin, U/ml	0,154
Total triiodothyronine level, nmol/l	0,135
Thyroid hormone level, mME/l	0,094
IgM level, mg/ml	0,074
1	**2**
IgA level, mg/ml	0,048
Level of total IgG autoantibodies to phospholipids, U/ml	0,041
Level of IgG-autoantibodies to [illegible]	0,012
Level of IgG autoantibodies to annexin V, units/ml	0,009
Cortisol level, nmol/l	0,006

Note: SCCDF values > 0.5 are marked in grey

Using these informative features, further cluster analysis of the laboratory parameters under study was performed. The most rational division into 3 clusters turned out to be, and the features characteristic of each cluster, as well as the presence of these features in the study groups are reflected in Table 10.

Table 10. Results of cluster processing informative blood indicators in Russian women

Informative indicators	**Centres cluster values**			**Correspondence of study groups to**		
	Cluster 1 n = 28	**Cluster 2 n = 27**	**Cluster 3 n = 26**	**Cluster 1**	**Cluster 2**	**Cluster 3**
Progesterone (nmol/l)	23,2	23,2	55,0	28 women with preserved reproductive health (Group 1)	27 women with reproductive health problems (Group 2)	26 women with reproductive health problems (Group 3)
Estradiol (pmol/l)	232,0	232,0	300,4			
Prolactin (mME/ml)	131,1	131,1	310,5			
Total thyroxine T4 (nmol/l)	85,2	85,2	124,9			
Autoantibodies to thyroglobulin	95,6	95,6	85,0			
TSTL, CD3+CD8+ (%)	18,2	21,4	18,2			
EQ, CD16+CD56+ (%)	12,0	15,1	12,0			
IgG-antibodies to β_2 -	3,2	5,0	3,2			

As follows from the table, the comparison of the values of informative indicators in different clusters showed that for the first 5 signs related to the hormonal status of women, clusters 1 and 2 fully coincided, but differed in these indicators from cluster 3. For the remaining 3 signs characterising immune status, clusters 1 and 3 coincided, but differed from cluster 2.

As a result, it turned out that the group of 28 healthy women (hereinafter referred to as group 1) fully corresponded to the quantitative values of cluster 1 in all tested indicators.

As for the group of 53 Russian women with pathological shifts in reproductive health, it was divided in the process of clustering into 2 subgroups of 27 and 26 people.

One of the subgroups (hereinafter group 2) completely corresponded to cluster 2 by the range of values of informative indicators and was characterised by differences in immunological indices. The second subgroup (hereinafter group 3) fully corresponded to cluster 3, which was characterised by the presence of peculiarities in the hormonal status.

Thus, from the standpoint of the ongoing study and according to the results of cluster analysis, among the 81 women selected for the study, it is reasonable to distinguish 3 study groups in the population of Russian women: (1) group 1 of 28 healthy women with preserved reproductive health; (2) group 2 with reproductive disorders presumably associated with abnormalities in immunological traits; (3) group 3 with reproductive disorders presumably associated with abnormalities in hormonal status.

In order to confirm the validity of the grouping and the assumptions made to assess its nature in the population of Russian women, the percentage of deviations of informative indicators in groups with impaired reproductive functions from those of healthy women was determined, as shown in Figure 14. .

The presented data fully confirm the fact that each formed group has pronounced statistically confirmed features, the clinical and physiological significance of which still requires further deciphering.

Special attention should be paid to the fact that in group 2 the most pronounced shifts are observed in immunological indicators - higher number of cells with cytotoxic activity (cytotoxic T-lymphocytes and natural killer cells), as well as higher content of IgG class antibodies to β2-glycoprotein. In group 3 with reproductive pathology, hormonal shifts prevail among the detected abnormalities of the indicators - higher blood content of estradiol and, especially, progesterone and prolactin, while the level of autoantibodies to thyroglobulin was lower than in women of the control group.

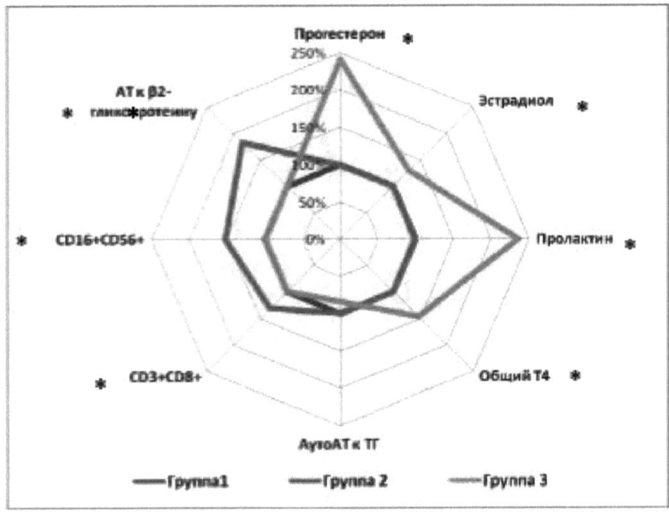

Figure 14: Percentage of deviation of informative indicators Russian women with reproductive pathologies from those with reproductive pathologies in healthy women

(* - differences between the values of indicators are statistically reliable)

To complete this piece of research, it would be desirable to determine whether there are differences between the subgroups at the genetic level, in particular in the presence of alleles characteristic of non-pregnancy.

The results of such genetic analyses for individual loci of genes controlling the immune response are presented in Figures 15-17.

Figure 15 shows that the HLA-DRB1 gene locus in healthy women in the Russian population is dominated by the allelic variant HLA-DRB1*12. In the presence of reproductive pathology, the greatest number of specific frequent alleles of this locus was observed in group 2 - HLA-DRB1*01, HLA-DRB1*04, HLA-DRB1*11, HLA-DRB1*13, and in group 3 the predominant alleles were HLA-DRB1*07 and HLA-DRB1*15 (the latter being favourable).

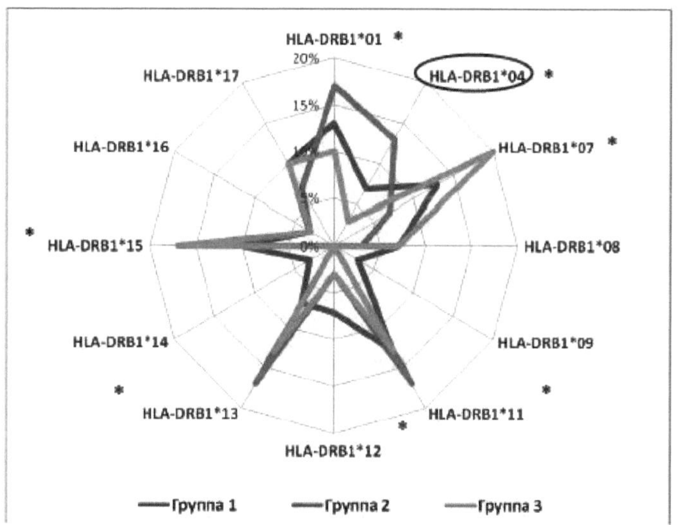

Figure 15: Frequency of occurrence of different alleles of the HLA-DRB1 locus in women of different groups in the Russian population
(* - differences between the values of the indicators are statistically reliable, oval alleles with unfavourable reproductive prognosis are marked)

Attention should be paid to the fact that in group 2, in which immunological abnormalities prevail, the unfavourable allele for miscarriage of pregnancy HLA-DRB1*04 is registered relatively often (in 13% of cases), while in control group 1 it occurs in 7.5% of cases

(1.7 times less frequently), and in risk group 3 - only in 3% of cases (4.3 times less frequently).

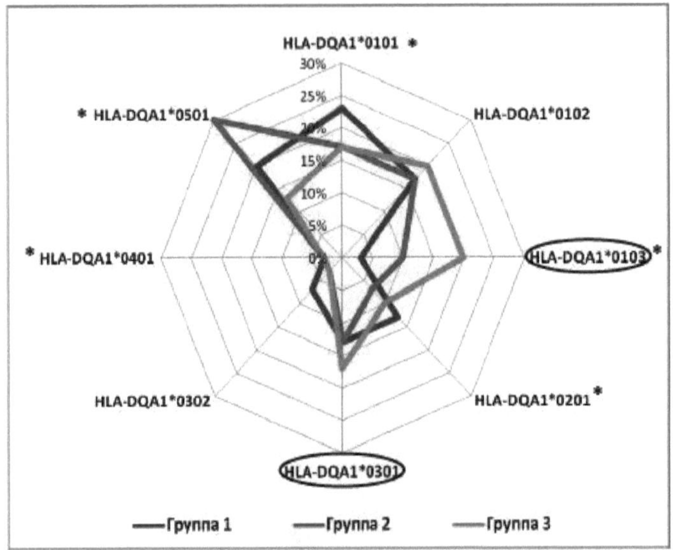

Figure 16: Frequency of occurrence of different alleles of the HLA-DQA1 locus in women of different groups in the Russian population

(* - differences between the values of the indicators are statistically reliable, oval alleles with unfavourable reproductive prognosis are marked)

When analysing allelic variants at the HLA-DQA1 locus, a different situation was noted (Figure 16).

The greatest diversity of alleles was characteristic of healthy women - HLA-DQA1*0101, HLA-DQA1*0201, HLA-DQA1*0302, of which the first two are considered favourable from the point of view of reproductive health and occur with a frequency of 23% and 13.5%, respectively.

In women with reproductive pathology, the prevalence of single alleles - HLA-DQA1*0501 in group 2 and HLA-DQA1*0103 in group 3 - was found. The HLA-DQA1*0103 allele is considered unfavourable and associated with foetal failure; it is registered in group 3, where the peculiarities of hormone nal status are noted, with a frequency of 20% (in every fifth woman), which is 2 times more frequent than in group 2 and 6.7 times more frequent than in the control group of women with preserved reproductive health.

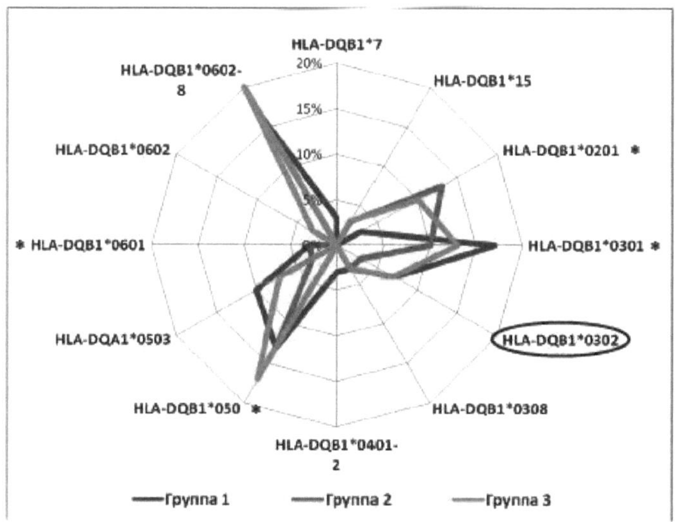

Figure 17: Frequency of occurrence of different alleles of the HLA-DQB1 locus in women of Russian populations

(* - differences between the values of the indicators are statistically reliable, oval alleles with unfavourable reproductive prognosis are marked)

A similar distribution was determined for the HLA-DQB1 locus (Figure 17). Two alleles - HLA-DQB1*0301 and HLA-DQB1*0503 - prevailed in healthy women, HLA-DQB1*0201 in women with reproductive pathology of group 2, and HLA-DQB1*050 in women with reproductive pathology of group 3, the association of which with reproductive disorders has not been previously noted. As for the HLA-DQB1*0302 allele, which is considered unfavourable from the point of view of its association with foetal abortion, it was registered in only 7% of women in both group 3 with a risk of reproductive disorders and group 1 with preserved reproductive function, and in group 2 with reproductive disorders based on immunological characteristics - only in 3% of cases.

Thus, according to the tested laboratory indicators, the studied population of Russian women, in addition to interpopulation differences, has a set of both genotypic and phenotypic features that can be used to assess the state of their reproductive health. Two categories of traits associated with reproductive disorders have been identified. One category concerns abnormalities in immune status and the second category concerns abnormalities in sex hormone levels. So far, it has also been established that both categories of abnormalities may, in principle, be genetic in nature, with abnormalities in immune status presumably associated with the presence of the HLA-DRB1*04 allele and abnormalities in sex hormones with carriage of the HLA-DQA1*0103 allele.

3.4 A cluster approach to reproductive health assessment Women living in the Faizabad district of Tajikistan

This section of the research analysed the relationship between selected laboratory criteria characterising genetic features, hormonal and immune status, and signs of antiphospholipid syndrome, and the reproductive health of women living in Tajikistan.

As in the case of the study of a population of Russian women, 85 women of reproductive age were monitored, of whom 28 had prenatal pregnancies that ended in the birth of healthy children (healthy women), and 57 had signs of reproductive health problems (pregnancy failure, premature births). The reproductive ive health of unborn women was not analysed in this research fragment.

Table 11. Standardised canonical coefficients of discriminant function of informative blood indicators in Tajik women with different reproductive health statuses

Informative blood counts	[SCCDF].
1	2
IgG-antibody level to β_2 -glycoprotein	3,879
Cortisol level (nmol/l)	3,326
Thyroperoxidase autoantibody level (IU/ml)	2,649
Total IgG-antibody level to phospholipids (IU/ml)	2,086
Estradiol level (pmol/l)	1,496
Prothrombin IgG antibody level (units/ml)	1,166
Prolactin level (mME/ml)	0,723
Total thyroxine T4 level (nmol/l)	0,528
Thyroglobulin autoantibody level (IU/ml)	0,508
Number of T-lymphocytes, CD3+ (%)	0,410
Progesterone level, nmol/l	0,272
Luteinising hormone level, IU/L	0,216
1	2
Lupus anticoagulant level, U/mL	0,216
Dihydroepiandrosterone sulphate level, nmol/L	0,193
17-OH progesterone level, nmol/L	0,187
Blood clotting time in lebetox test, min.	0,175
Number of T-helper cells, CD3+CD4+ (%)	0,153
Level of IgG-antibodies to annexin V (units/ml)	0,153
Thyroid hormone level, mME/l	0,132
Number of natural killer cells, CD16+CD56+ (%)	0,133
Number of cytotoxic T-lymphocytes, CD3+CD8+ (%)	0,127
Number of ECTs, CD3+CD56+ (%)	0,125
Testosterone level, nmol/l	0,123
IgG level, mg/ml	0,117
IgA level, mg/ml	0,110
Total triiodothyronine level, nmol/l	0,104

Follicle stimulating hormone level, IU/L	0,095
IgM level, mg/ml	0,083
Number of B-lymphocytes, CD19+ (%)	0,010

Note: SCCDF values > 0.5 are marked in grey

The sign of preserved or impaired reproductive health was used as the basis for discriminant analysis. Nine informative indicators of such a distinction, ranked by the value of the SCCDF, are presented in Table 11. As in the population of Russian women, values of the coefficient above 0.5 were taken as the conditional value of the SCCDF at which a trait was considered highly informative.

As follows from the discriminant analysis, the set of the most informative indicators of reproductive health and the results of their ranking in Tajik women is fundamentally different from that in Russian women. While in the latter case the most significant were the levels of thyroc syn and oestradiol hormones, as well as the blood content of natural killer cells and cyto toxic T-lymphocytes, in the Tajik population the leading place was occupied by the levels of cortisol, oestradiol, progesterone, prolactin and the levels of various autoantibodies, including those determining the development of antiphos foli pide reactions.

Further, cluster analysis of the laboratory indicators under study was carried out, the results of which are shown in Table 12. Similarly to the Russian population, for Tajik women the most rational division into 3 clusters and, accordingly, the allocation of 3 study groups turned out to be the most rational.

As follows from the table, by the first 6 indicators, which characterise the hormonal status to some extent, clusters 1 and 3 coincide completely, while cluster 2 has a certain peculiarity: the first three indicators were lower, and the following three indicators took higher values.

Table 12. Results of cluster processing informative blood parameters in Tajik women

Informative indicators	Centres cluster values			Correspondence of study groups to		
	Cluster 1	Cluster 2	Cluster 3	Cluster 1	Cluster 2	Cluster 3
Estradiol (pmol/l)	249,7	230,3	249,7	28 women with preserved reproductive health (group 1)	27 women with impaired reproductive health (group 2)	29 women with impaired reproductive health (group 3)
Prolactin (mME/ml)	209,8	125,1	209,8			
Total thyroxine T4 (nmol/l)	100,3	79,9	100,3			
Autoantibodies to thyroglobulin (IU/ml)	54,3	84,3	54,3			
Autoantibodies to thyroperoxidase	23,8	45,5	23,8			
Cortisol (nmol/l)	250,4	340,2	250,4			
IgG-antibodies to human phospholipids	6,5	6,5	9,6	28 women with preserved reproductive health (group 1)	28 women with reproductive disorders (group 2)	29 women with reproductive disorders (group 2)
IgG-antibodies to β_2 - glycoprotein	7,2	7,1	10,0			
IgG-antibodies to prothrombin (units/ml)	6,6	10,0	10,0			

For the last three informative indicators associated with antiphospholipid reaction, each cluster was characterised by peculiarities, with all 28 women with preserved reproductive function falling into cluster 1 (hereinafter group 5). This cluster was characterised by the ranges of values of all informative indicators within the conventional physiological norm (ref rence values). Half of the women with impaired reproductive health corresponded to cluster 2 (hereinafter group 6), and the remaining women with unfavourable obstetric history corresponded to cluster 3 (hereinafter group 7).

The nature of deviations in the ranges of values of indicators for reproductive health disorders in women of the Tajik population is particularly illustrated in Figure 18.

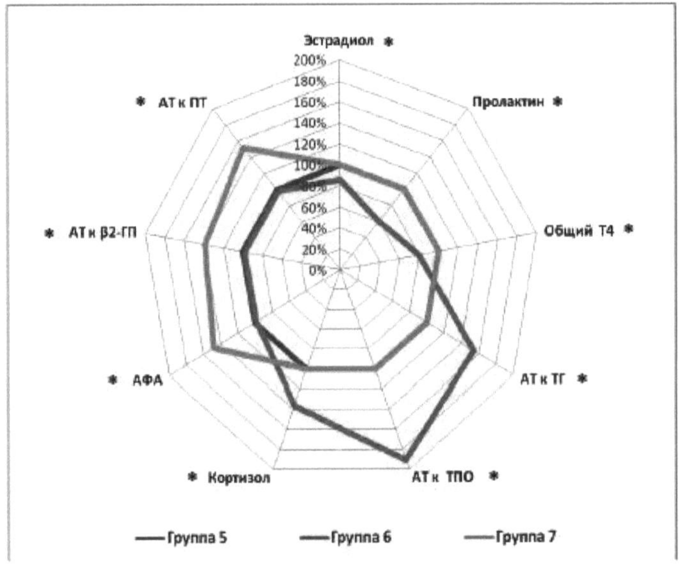

Figure 18: Percentage of deviation of informative indicators Tajik women with reproductive pathology from those with reproductive pathology in reproductively healthy women

(* - differences between the values of indicators are statistically reliable)

The figure shows the percentage of deviations of data in clusters 5 and 6 (reproductive pathology) from those in cluster 1 (healthy women). Cluster 5, to which half of the women with reproductive disorders belong, differs rather unfavourably, with a decrease in the level of informative sex hormones and one of their thyroid hormones, an increase in the level of cortisol, and a selective increase in autoantibodies to thyroid proteins. Another part of women with reproductive disorders from cluster 6 is characterised by selective growth of IgG-antibodies to phospholipids, β_2 -glycoprotein and prothrombin.

As follows from the data obtained, the very cluster principle of data grouping in the populations of Russian and Tajik women roughly coincides: (1) there is a separate control group of women with preserved reproductive health, (2) the group with reproductive disorders in the anamnesis is divided into two approximately equal subgroups.

At the same time, the set of information features in each population under consideration differs significantly from each other, which affects, first of all, the features of groups with reproductive disorders. Thus, in Russian women, the cluster principle allows us to distinguish a group with peculiarities of the cellular-phenotypic composition of immunograms (group 2), as well as single autoimmune abnormalities, and a group with peculiarities of the hormonal status in the direction of an increase in the content of sex hormones and individual thyroid hormones (group 3). In women of Tajik population among the category with unfavourable obstetric anamnesis it was possible to identify a group with deviations in hormonal status in the direction of a decrease in sex hormones and thyroxine in the blood with an increase in autoantibodies to thyroid components and cortisol levels (group 6), as well as a group with shifts in the content of autoantibodies in the direction of antiphospholipid reaction (group 7).

Further, allelic variants of individual loci of genes controlling immune response were studied in Tajik women (Figures 19-21).

Figure 19 shows that the HLA-DRB1 gene locus in healthy women of the Tajik population is dominated by the HLA-DRB1*17 allele variant, while the HLA-DRB1*12 allele was more common in Russian women than in other groups.

In the presence of reproductive pathology, the greatest number of specific frequent alleles of the indicated locus was observed in group 6 - HLA-DRB1*01, HLA-DRB1*04, HLA-DRB1*13, and as in the population of Russian women, while in group 6 the predominant alleles were HLA-DRB1*11 and HLA-DRB1*15 (the former as in group 2, and the latter as in group 3 in Russian women). The HLA-DRB1*04 allele, as already mentioned, was associated with reproductive disorders, and the HLA-DRB1*15 allele was associated with prote to ical properties. The frequency of occurrence of the unfavourable HLA-DRB1*04 allele in group 6 was 13%, as in the population of Russian women.

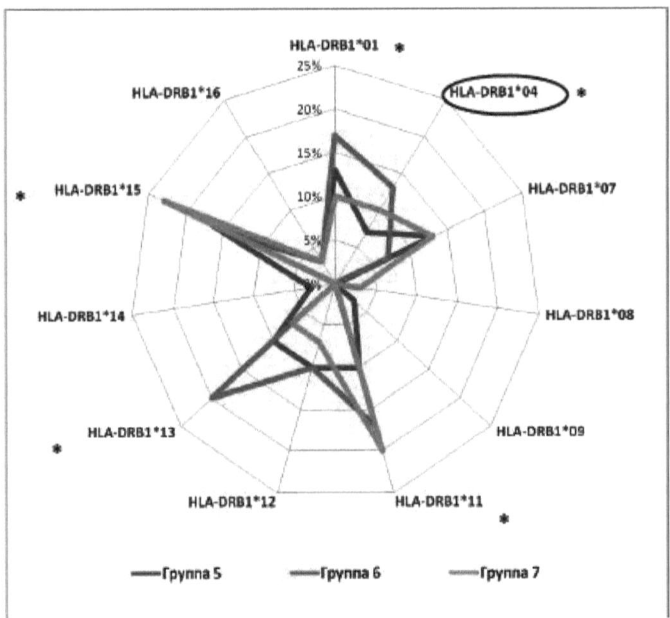

Figure 19: Frequency of occurrence of different alleles of the HLA-DRB1 locus in women of different groups in the Tajik population

(* - differences between the values of the indicators are statistically reliable, oval alleles with unfavourable reproductive prognosis are marked)

Thus, allelic differences have been detected at the HLA-DRB1 locus in healthy women of the Russian and Tajik populations, but in women with reproductive disorders, regardless of group affiliation, the set of allelic variants in general coincides completely.

The results of the analysis of allelic variants at the HLA-DQA1 locus are shown in Figure 20. Reproductively healthy women were characterised by the prevalence of HLA-DQA1*0102 alleles (a favourable allele characteristic of reproductive health) and HLA-DQA1*0301 (in Russian women - HLA-DQA1*0101, HLA-DQA1*0201, HLA-DQA1*0302).

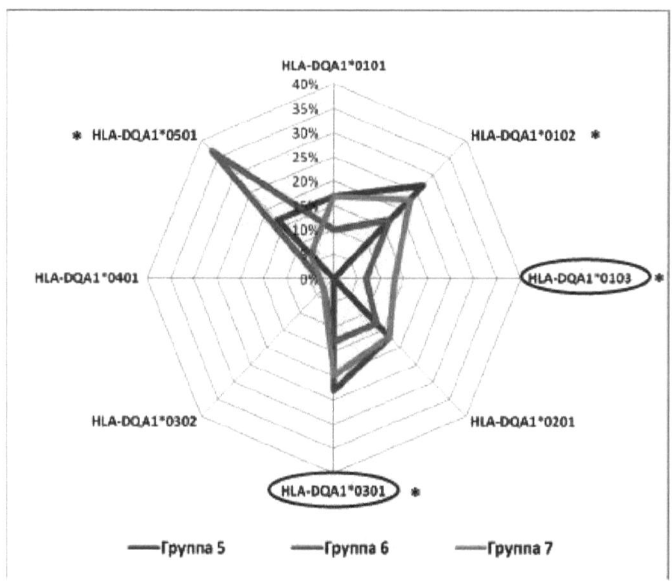

Figure 20: Frequency of occurrence of different alleles of the HLA-DQA1 locus in women of different groups in the Tajik population

(* - differences between the values of the indicators are statistically reliable, oval alleles with unfavourable reproductive prognosis are marked)

HLA-DQA1*0501 allele was most frequently registered in Tajik women with reproductive pathology in group 6 and HLA-DQA1*0103 allele in group 7. The latter allele is considered unfavourable and associated with pregnancy failure, and its frequency of occurrence in the Tajik population was 13.5%, i.e. 1.5 times less frequent than in the Russian population, but with approximately the same frequency of occurrence in other study groups as in Russian women.

The frequency of the HLA-DQA1*0301 allele, which is unfavourable for pregnancy failure, in the Tajik population deserves special comment. This allele was most often registered in women with preserved reproductive function (in 23.5% of cases), but with approximately the same frequency (20% of cases) it was found in women with impaired reproductive function in group 7. This fact once again demonstrates that not always the carriage of an unfavourable allelic variant of the named gene lecus can be realised in the form of reproductive health disorders, but the impact of external factors and phenotypic conditions in which a woman develops pregnancy are also important.

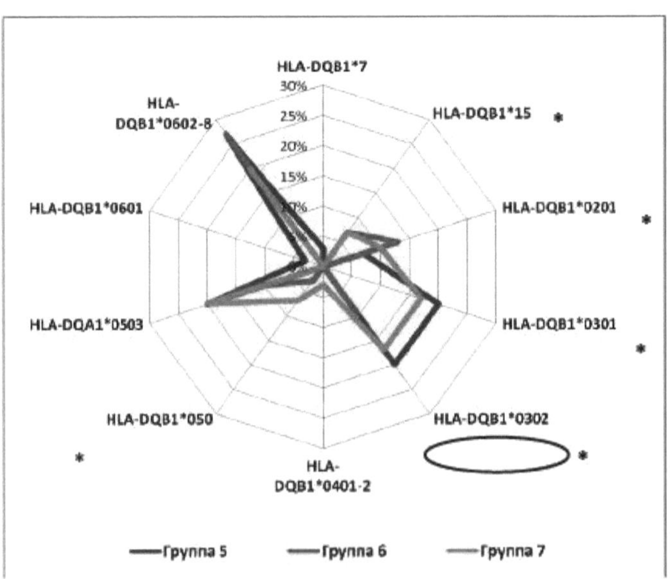

Figure 21: Frequency of occurrence of different alleles of the HLA-DQB1 locus in women of different groups in the Tajik population
(* - differences between the values of the indicators are statistically reliable, oval
alleles with unfavourable reproductive prognosis are marked)

When analysing the HLA-DQB1 locus (Figure 21), it was found that in healthy Tajik women the HLA-DQB1*0301 and HLA-DQB1*0302 alleles prevailed (in Russian women - HLA-DQB1*0301 and HLA-DQB1*0503). The HLA-DQB1*0201 (group 6) and HLA-DQB1*050 (group 7) alleles were more frequent in Tajik women with reproductive pathology than in other cases, as well as in similar groups of the Russian population of women. The unfavourable allele HLA-DQB1*0302 with approximately equal frequency was observed in the control group (in 20% of cases) and in group 7 with reproductive disorders (in 17% of cases).

Thus, genetic studies on the allele frequency of a number of loci of genes controlling the immune response have revealed a number of interesting patterns. In the populations of Russian and Tajik women with preserved reproductive function, there is a rather pronounced diversity of allelic variants of HLA-DRB1, HLA-DQA1, and HLA-DQB1 loci, with the possibility of occurrence of unfavourable allelic variants. At the same time, women with reproductive disorders had the same alleles of the above loci, including those unfavourable for pregnancy failure, the set of which, as a rule, did not depend on the woman's belonging to the Russian or Tajik population.

Summary to chapter 3

1. When analysing the reproductive health of women belonging to different ethnic groups and living in regions with special climatic tic conditions, it is advisable to form separate physiological gi cial norms (reference values) of the laboratory indicators under study.

2. There are differences between the populations of Russian and Tajik women in a number of parameters of hormonal and immune status, as well as at the level of allelic variants of genes controlling the immune response, which should be taken into account when assessing the reproductive health of women belonging to these populations. .

2. On the basis of cluster-population analysis, a rational way of grouping the studied contingents of women of reproductive age was established to identify prenozological criteria of reproductive dysfunction. .

3. Two categories of factors associated with reproductive pathology have been identified in both women living in the Middle Black Earth Region of Russia and women living in the Faizabad District of Tajikistan.

4. The factors associated with impaired female reproductive functions include a set of genotypic differences in the presence of certain allelic variants of HLA-DRB1, HLA-DQA1, and HLA-DQB1 loci of genes responsible for the immune response, especially such alleles as HLA-DRB1*04 and HLA-DQA1*103 associated with pregnancy failure in both populations.

5. In the study of populations of Russian and Tajik women using the method of cluster-population analysis, it was confirmed that pathology of repro duction can in principle be associated with changes in several groups of factors - blood levels of sex hormones, the state of thyroid function, blood levels of cortisol, features of phenotypic composition of lymphocytes, and the presence of signs of antiphospholipid reaction.

CHAPTER 4. HORMONAL STATUS AND RISK GROUPS FOR REPRODUCTIVE HEALTH DISORDERS IN WOMEN

4.1 Hormonal status and risk groups for disorders Reproductive health of women in the Russian population

The main objective of this section of the research was to identify risk markers of reproductive health disorders among the indicators characterising the hormonal status of women in the Russian population. Such indicators included the levels of sex hormones in the blood, the content of pituitary and ovarian sex hormones in the blood, thyroid and adrenal hormones, and the levels of autoantibodies to thyroid hormones.

4.1.1 Sex hormones and risk groups for disorders Reproductive function in Russian women

It was found that among 107 women in the Russian population there is a contingent of 26 people (group 3) in whom reproductive disorders are associated with abnormalities in blood levels of sex hormones. The objective of this section of the study was to determine the nature of these abnormalities and to develop on their basis possible markers of such disorders at the prenosological stage.

Within the framework of this study the blood content of the following sex hormones was studied: pituitary hormones - follicle-stimulating hormone (FSH), luteinising hormone (LH), prolactin; ovarian hormones - estradiol, progesterone and the latter's metabolite 17-OH-progesterone (17-OP); androgens - testosterone and its metabolite dihydroepiandrosterone (DHEA-C).

The content of sex hormones was analysed according to the population-cluster principle in the following study groups: (1) group 1 - women of the Russian population with preserved reproductive function; (2) group 2 - women of the Russian population with reproductive disorders and predominance of immunological shifts; (3) group 3 - women of the Russian population with reproductive disorders and predominance of hormonal shifts.

The results of the study of sex hormone levels in the blood of women in the Russian population grouped according to the above principle are presented in Table 13 and Figure 22.

Table 13. Sex hormone levels in women of the Russian population in the study groups

Informative indicators	Median indicator [minimum, maximum]			p_1 p_2 p_3
	Group 1	Group 2	Group 3	
FSH (IU/L)	4,0 [1,3; 7,5]	4,0 [1,1; 7,7]	5,3 [3,4; 6,6]	0,893 0,023 0,019
LH (IU/L)	4,0 [2,7; 5,9]	4,3 [1,7; 7,6]	6,4 [5,1; 8,5]	0,443 <0,001 <0,001
Prolactin (mME/ml)	131,6 [126,4; 134,1]	131,6 [126,4; 136,0]	308,7 [300,7; 321,0]	0,893 <0,001 <0,001
Estradiol (pmol/l)	232,4 [227,9; 236,3]	232,9 [228,0; 240,0]	300,2 [297,2; 302,4]	0,469 <0,001 <0,001
Progesterone (nmol/l)	22,6 [19,1; 29,3]	22,7 [19,1; 50,3]	55,0 [52,4; 56,7]	0,827 <0,001 <0,001
17-OP (nmol/l)	2,8 [0,4; 6,6]	2,8 [0,7; 6,2]	2,6 [0,2; 6,0]	0,973 0,612 0,621
Testosterone (nmol/l)	2,6 [0,2; 6,6]	2,2 [0,5; 6,0]	1,6 [0,5; 3,0]	0,813 0,055 0,028
DHEAS (nmol/l)	3,8 [2,6; 6,4]	3,9 [2,9; 6,2]	3,6 [2,1; 6,2]	0,538 0,052 0,079

Note: p_1 - probability of differences between groups 1 and 2; p_2 - probability of differences between groups 2 and 3; p_3 - probability of differences between groups 1 and 3; grey indicates the significance of differences ($p<0.05$) according to the Mann-Whitney test.

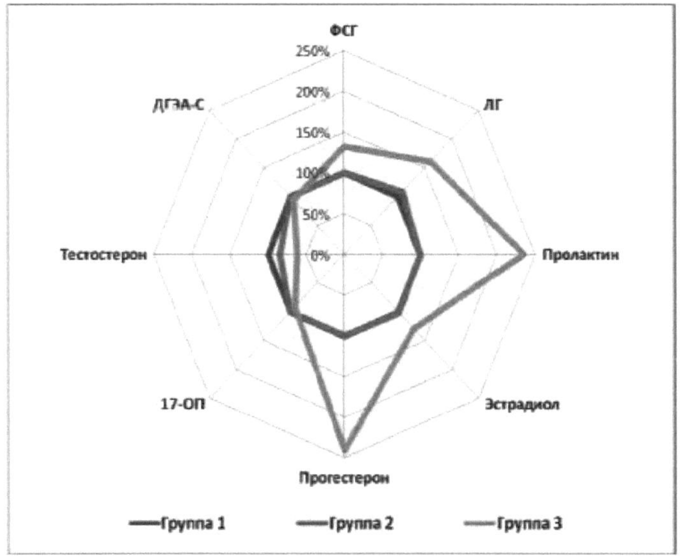

Figure 22: Percentages of deviation of sex hormone levels in Russian women with reproductive disorders from those of healthy women

(* - differences between the values of indicators are statistically reliable)

The data obtained show that the nature of deviations in the content of sex hormones in the blood of women in the Russian population at risk for reproductive disorders is ambiguous.

As has been shown earlier, of the two risk groups identified by cluster analysis, only one (group 3) showed a significant increase in the blood levels of follicle-stimulating hormone, luteinising hormone, prolactin, estradiol and progesterone, which occurs against the background of a significant decrease in testosterone levels. In the other risk group (group 2), the indicators of sex hormone content almost completely correspond to those of healthy women.

Next, we tested all the named hormones with statistically significant deviations in risk group 3 as markers of hormonal abnormalities in the respective group. To this end, we first determined the 95% confidence intervals of each of the named hormones in the respective study group to determine the range of values in which statistically significant deviations occur, and then established the degree of their prognostic significance.

Prognostic significance was determined by constructing a ROC-curve reflecting the state of linear regression between sensitivity and specificity of the diagnostic test, followed by calculation of the area under the ROC-curve - AUROC. In modern scientific literature, AUROC is quite widely used to confirm the diagnostic significance of various tests: with AUROC values below 0.6 the test is not considered diagnostically significant, in the range of 0.6-0.8 the test shows moderate diagnostic significance, and with AUROC values above 0.8 the diagnostic significance of the test is considered quite high with the maximum AUROC value equal to 1.0 [80, 219, 342].

Figures 23-28 show the 95% confidence intervals (95% CI) and predictive value of the tests for the level of each informative sex hormone in a population of Russian women.

Thus, Figure 23 on the left shows the 95% confidence intervals for the level of follicle-stimulating hormone. As can be seen from the graph, the ranges of values of this indicator are very close to each other and, despite the fact that these values are slightly higher for Russian women in group 3, but still most of the values in the groups overlap. The AUROC value of 0.707 shows that this indicator shows only moderate prognostic significance when comparing different groups.

Figure 23. 95% confidence intervals of follicle-stimulating hormone levels in the blood of Russian women of the studied groups and ROC-curve of the predictive value of the test
(pink colour indicates the reference value area)

Thus, the statistical technique based on the determination of 95% confidence intervals of the indicators and the construction of ROC-curve allows us to consider that the level of pituitary follicle-stimulating hormone can hardly claim to be a test with high prognostic significance in the population of Russian women.

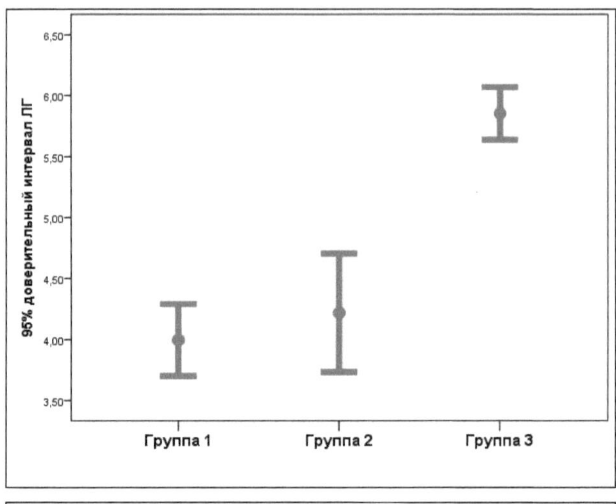

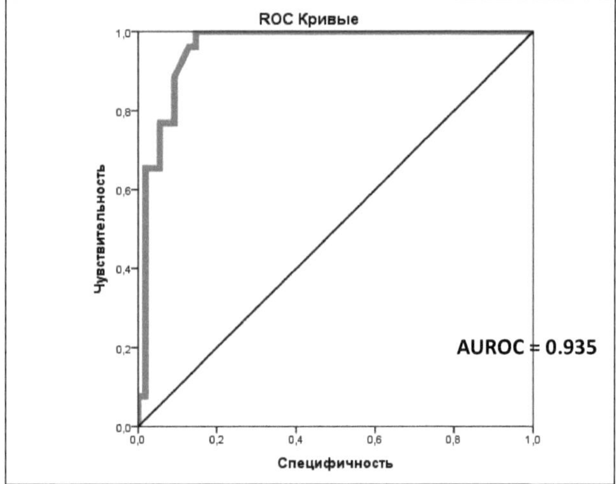

Figure 24. 95% confidence intervals of luteinising lutein levels hormone in the blood of Russian women of the studied groups and ROC-curve of the predictive value of the test

(pink colour indicates the reference value area)

Figure 24 shows graphical representations of the results of determining the range of values and prognostic significance of another pituitary hormone, luteinising hormone. As the graph shows, in Russian women the level of luteinising hormone was higher in risk group 3, with a high predictive value of this indicator (AUROC = 0.959), when its value was approximately higher than 4.8 IU/l.

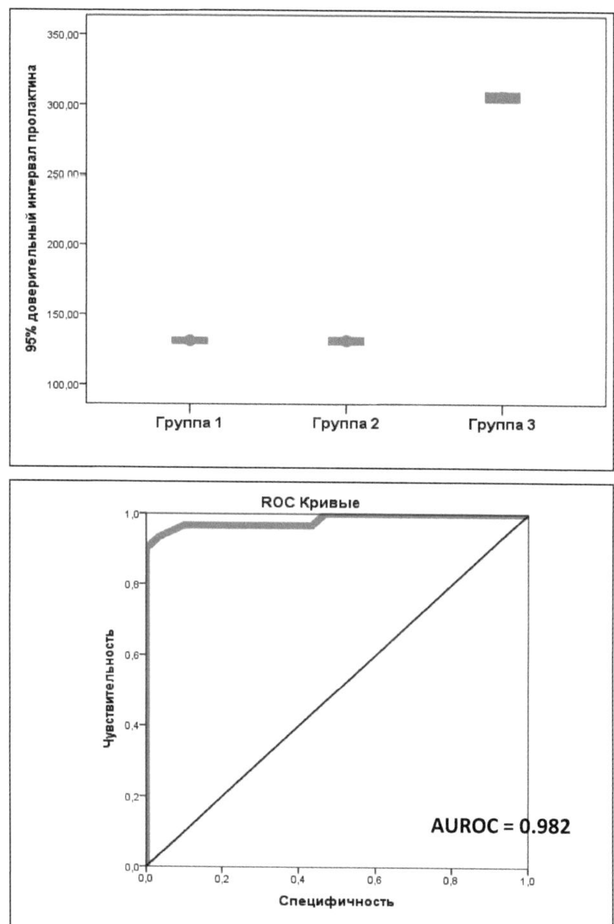

Figure 25. 95% confidence intervals of prolactin levels in the blood of Russian women of the studied groups and ROC curve of the predictive value of the test

(pink colour indicates the reference value area)

Figure 25 clearly shows that the level of another pituitary hormone, prolactin, is a fairly reliable prognostic sign that women in the Russian population belong to the risk group for reproductive

Tajik women

disorders (group 3). In this group, the prognostically significant prolactin values were in the range of values approximately above 300 mIU/ml, and the AUROC value was very high - 0.982.

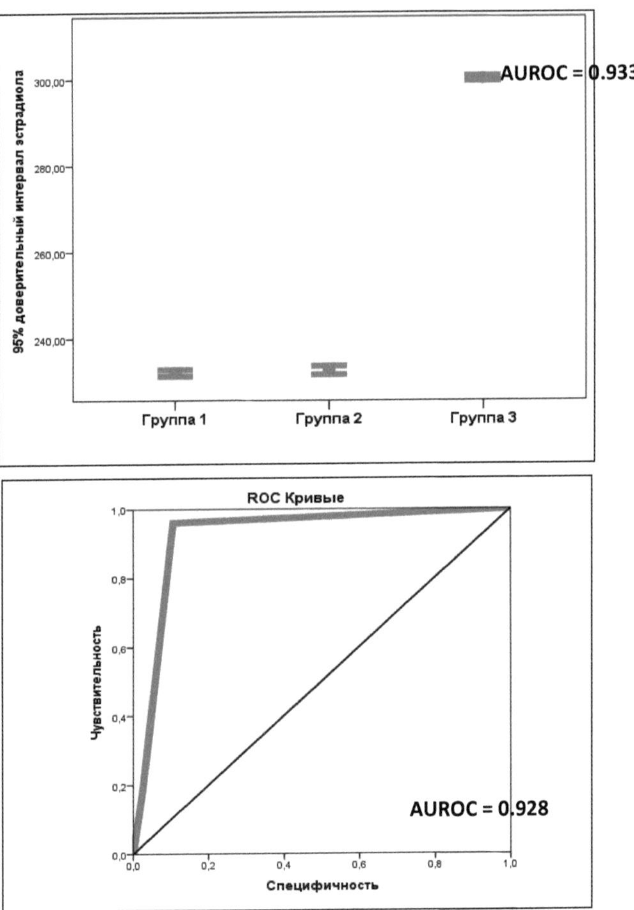

Figure 26. 95% confidence intervals of estradiol levels in the blood of Russian women of the studied groups and ROC-curve of the predictive value of the test

(pink colour indicates the reference value area)

Ovarian hormones, in particular oestradiol, were also found to have a high predictive value, as presented in Figure 26. Like many other sex hormones, the 95% confidence interval of estradiol was significantly higher in the group of 3 Russian women (approximately above 290 pmol/l). The prognostic significance of these deviations was very high, as the value of the area under the ROC curve (AUROC) approached the maximum and reached 0.928.

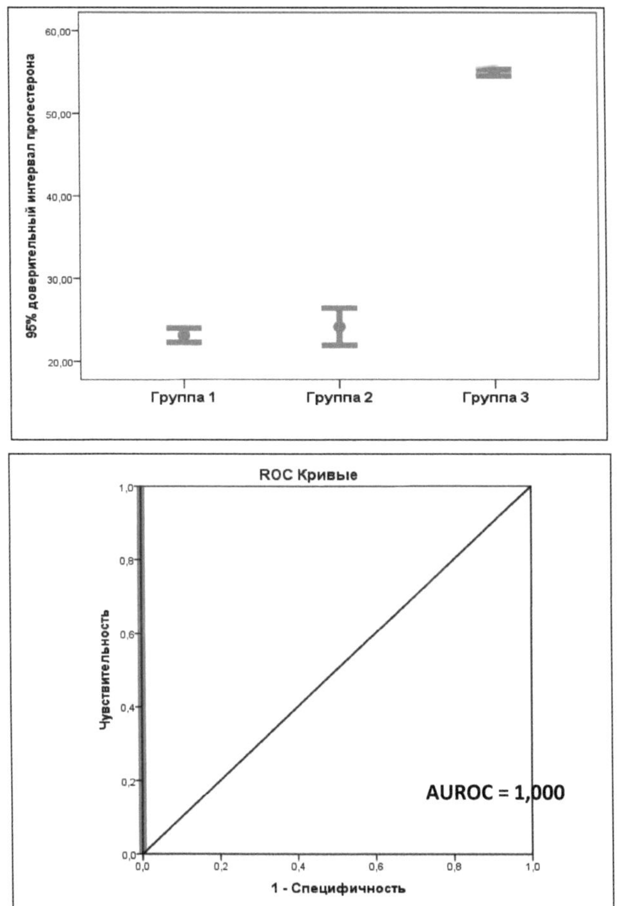

Figure 27. 95% confidence intervals of progesterone levels in the blood of Russian women of the study groups and ROC curve of the predictive value of the test

(pink colour indicates the reference value area)

Another important ovarian hormone, progesterone, was also highly predictive (AUROC took maximum values and was 1,000), as shown in Figure 27. In the Russian population, its content approximately above 50 nmol/l allowed to assign a woman to the risk group (in our study, group 3).

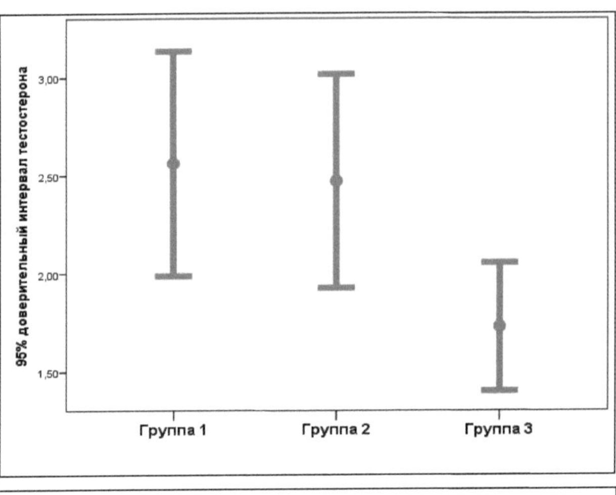

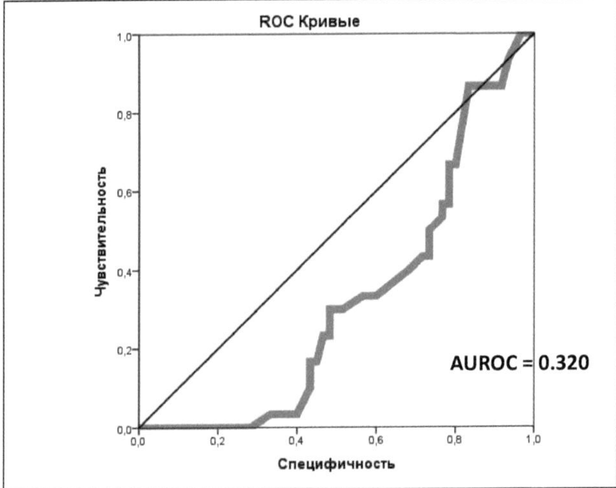

Figure 28. 95% confidence intervals of testosterone levels in the blood of Russian women of the study groups and ROC curve the predictive value of the test

(pink colour indicates the reference value area)

The biologically inactive metabolite of progesterone - 17-OH-progesterone - can serve as a source of testosterone formation in the body, but it cannot claim to be a marker of reproductive disorders in women of the Russian population, as well as the metabolite of testosterone - dihydroepiandrosterone. For them, 95% confidence intervals for group data and ROC-curve construction were not performed, as they did not show reliable intergroup differences.

Figure 28 shows the results of assessing the prognostic role of testosterone, a male sex hormone (androgen) produced in the female body by the ovaries and adrenal glands. This hormone can hardly claim to be a marker of reproductive disorders in Russian women, as its 95% confidence intervals in different groups overlapped, and the AUROC value was rather low and was only 0.320.

Thus, the studies in this section have confirmed that the pathogenesis of reproductive disorders in Russian women may be based on shifts in blood levels of sex hormones. In a part of the Russian population of women belonging to group 3 and having, judging by the obstetric history, signs of risk of reproductive disorders, these shifts were most often manifested by an increase in the production of female sex hormones in the pituitary gland and ovaries and a decrease in the level of androgens, most often produced in the ovaries. However, a more detailed statistical analysis showed that, despite this, only a small group of sex hormones can serve as a marker of the risk group for the development of reproductive disorders. Luteinising hormone, prolactin, estradiol and progesterone belonged to this category of marker hormones.

4.1.2 Thyroid and adrenal hormones and groups risk of women's reproductive health risks Russian population

It is known that, in addition to sex hormones, the state of hormonal function of such endocrine organs as the thyroid gland and adrenal glands can affect the state of the reproductive system in women. Autoimmune process may be one of the mechanisms of such disorder. In this regard, this section of research is devoted to the study of the role of thyroid and adrenal hormones in the development of reproductive pathology from the perspective of the population cluster approach.

The results of such a study in a population of Russian women divided into groups (clusters) based on obstetric history are presented in Table 14 and Figure 29. The objects of the study in this case were the blood levels of the following hormones: thyroid hormone, total triiodothyronine (T3), total thyroxine (T4), and cortisol. In addition, as already mentioned, thyroid function in the female organism, including that associated with pregnancy failure, could be affected by the accumulation of autoantibodies to thyroid proteins - thyroglobulin and thyroperoxidase enzyme, the assessment of which was also included in this fragment of the study.

As follows from the presented data, the level of thyroid hormones, autoantibodies to thyroid components, and cortisol changes to a significant extent in a part of women with reproductive disorders. Thus, in women of the Russian population belonging to group 3 according to the cluster analysis, there is a significant increase in the levels of thyroid hormones with a significant decrease in the levels of autoantibodies to thyroid proteins and cortisol.

Table 14. Hormonal status in women of the Russian population by study group

Informative indicators	Median indicator [minimum,			p_1 p_2 p_3
	Group 1	Group 2	Group 3	

Thyroid hormone (mME/l)	0,45 [0,1; 1,8]	0,4 [0,1; 1,7]	2,6 [0,5; 5,2]	0,604 <0,001 <0,001
Total T3 (nmol/ml)	1,5 [0,1; 3,1]	1,5 [0,1; 2,6]	2,4 [0,1; 7,0]	0,787 0,005 0,008
Total T4 (nmol/l)	85,3 [83,0; 90,0]	85,0 [83,0; 90,0]	125,4 [119,2; 127,2]	0,742 <0,001 <0,001
Autoantibodies to thyroglobulin (IU/ml)	4,8 [4,65; 4,95]	4,8 [4,65; 4,90]	4,2 [4,15; 4,50]	0,808 <0,001 <0,001
Autoantibodies to thyroperoxidase (IU/ml)	25,1 [23,9; 26,0]	25,1 [24,0; 25,8]	20,1 [19,1; 21,0]	0,966 <0,001 <0,001
Cortisol (nmol/l)	320,0 [317,0; 360,0]	320,0 [317,4; 350,0]	209,9 [207,4; 212,3]	0,827 <0,001 <0,001

Note: p_1 - probability of differences in groups 1 and 2; p_2 - probability of differences in groups 2 and 3; p_3 - probability of differences in data in groups 1 and 3; grey indicates the significance of differences ($p<0.05$) by the Mann-Whitney test

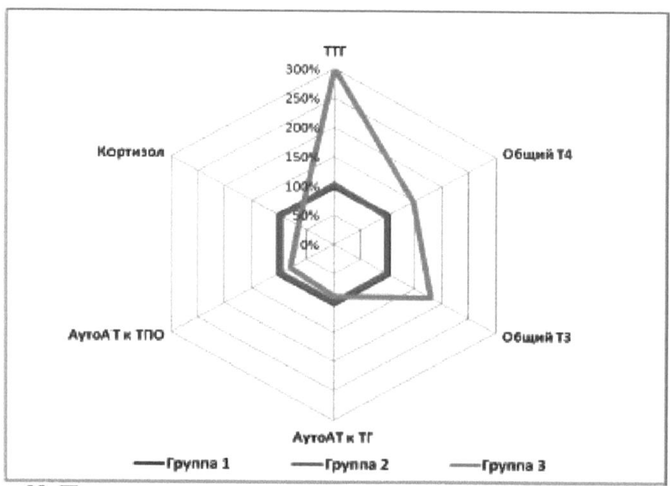

Fig. 29. Percentages of deviation of hormonal status indicators in women with reproductive disorders compared to healthy women

(* - differences between the values of indicators are statistically reliable)

To address the question of what changes in thyroid and adrenal functions may serve as markers of reproductive disorders in these groups of women in the Russian population, the data were analysed for prognostic significance. For this purpose, 95% confidence intervals were determined for each indicator in each group and a ROC-curve was constructed with calculation of the AUROC value. These data are presented in Figures 30-35.

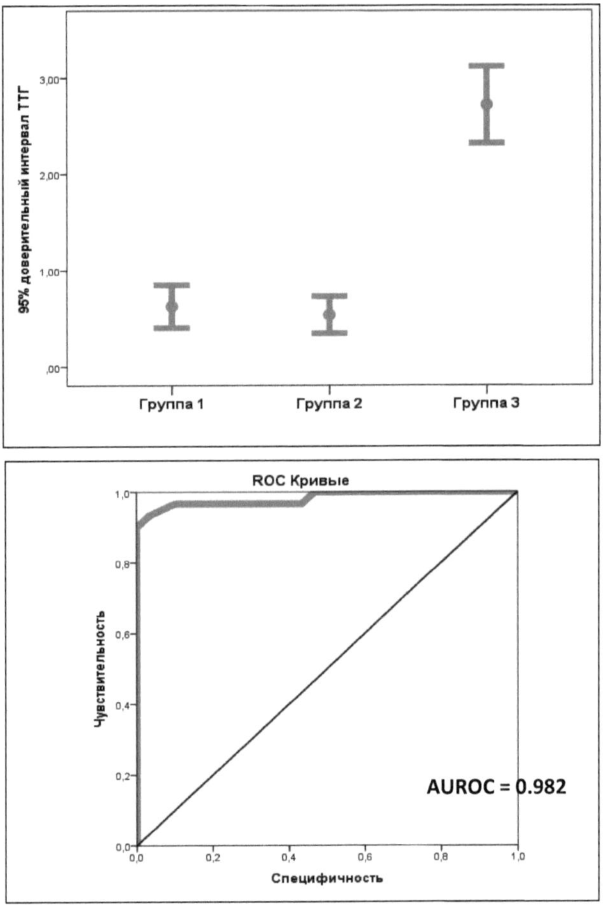

Figure 30. 95% confidence intervals of thyroid hormone levels in the blood of Russian women of the study groups and ROC curve the predictive value of the test
(pink colour indicates the reference value area)

Figure 30 shows 95% confidence intervals of thyroid hormone levels in different groups of women belonging to the Russian population. Group 3 women showed 95% confidence intervals in the range of values approximately above 1.7 mIU/L, which is significantly higher than in the other groups, with a high predictive value of this indicator (AUROC = 0.982).

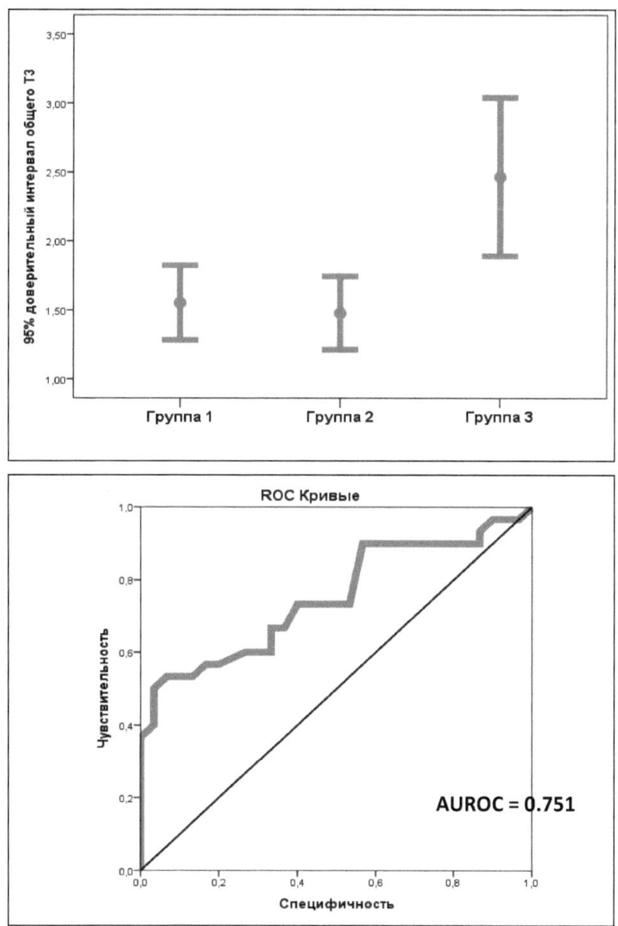

Figure 31. 95% confidence intervals of total triiodothyronine levels

in the blood of Russian women of the study groups and ROC curve
the predictive value of the test
(pink colour indicates the reference value area)

As Figure 31 shows, the content of total triiodothyronine in the blood can hardly claim to be a marker of possible reproductive disorders, since in the population of Russian women this indicator showed only moderate prognostic significance, which, in the presence of indicators with high prognostic significance, makes the use of this test inappropriate.

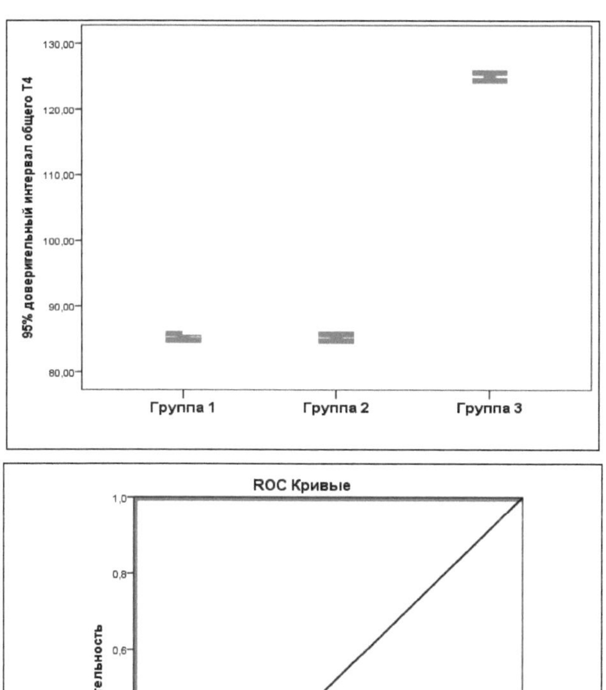

Figure 32. 95% confidence intervals of total thyroxine levels in the blood of Russian women of the study groups and ROC curve the predictive value of the test

(pink colour indicates the reference value area)

The level of total thyroxine in the blood of women in the Russian population (Figure 32), with values approximately above 100 nmol/l, indicated that the woman belonged to a risk group (group 3) for reproductive health disorders, with an absolute prognostic value, judging by the AUROC value of 1.0.

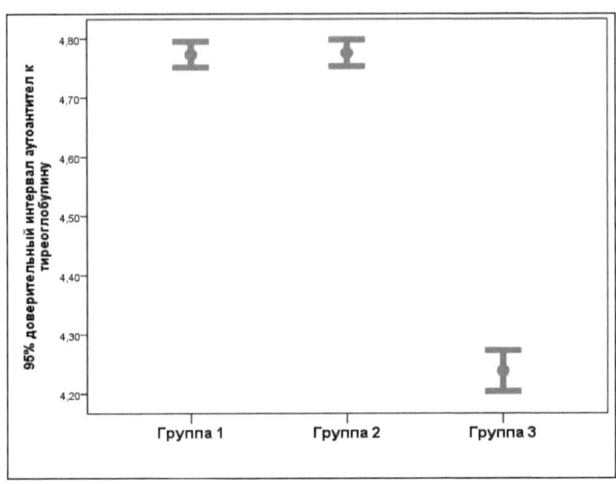

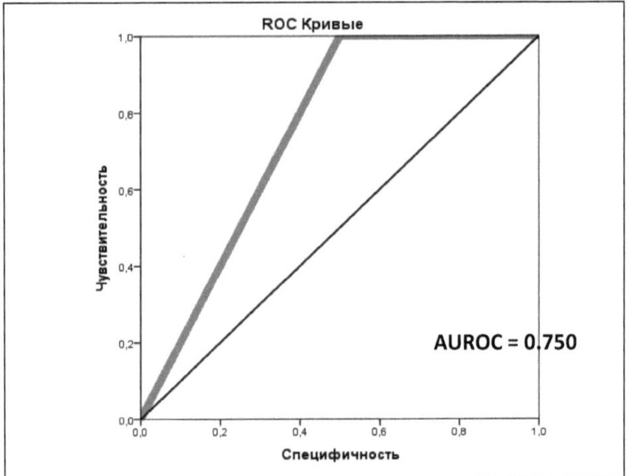

Figure 33. 95% confidence intervals of thyroglobulin autoantibody levels in the blood of Russian women in the study groups and ROC curves of the predictive value of the test
(pink colour indicates the reference value area)

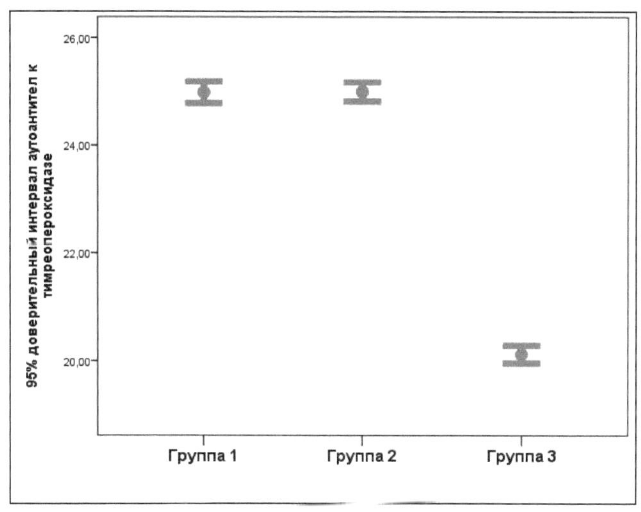

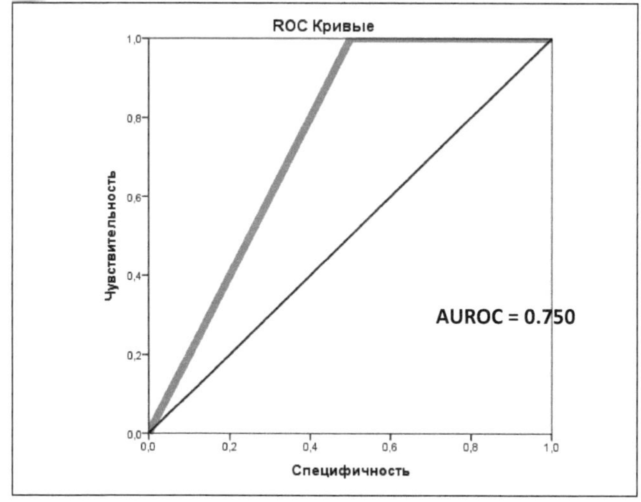

Figure 34. 95% confidence intervals of levels of autoantibodies to thyroperoxidase in the blood of Russian women of the study groups and ROC curves of the predictive value of the test
(pink colour indicates the reference value area)

In the population of Russian women, the 95% confidence interval of autoantibody levels to thyroglobulin (Figure 33) and to thyroperoxidase (Figure 34) in risk group 3 was lower than in other groups, judging from the figures. However, analysis of the prognostic significance of these tests showed that it is moderate and, therefore, limited in its use as markers of the risk of reproductive health disorders.

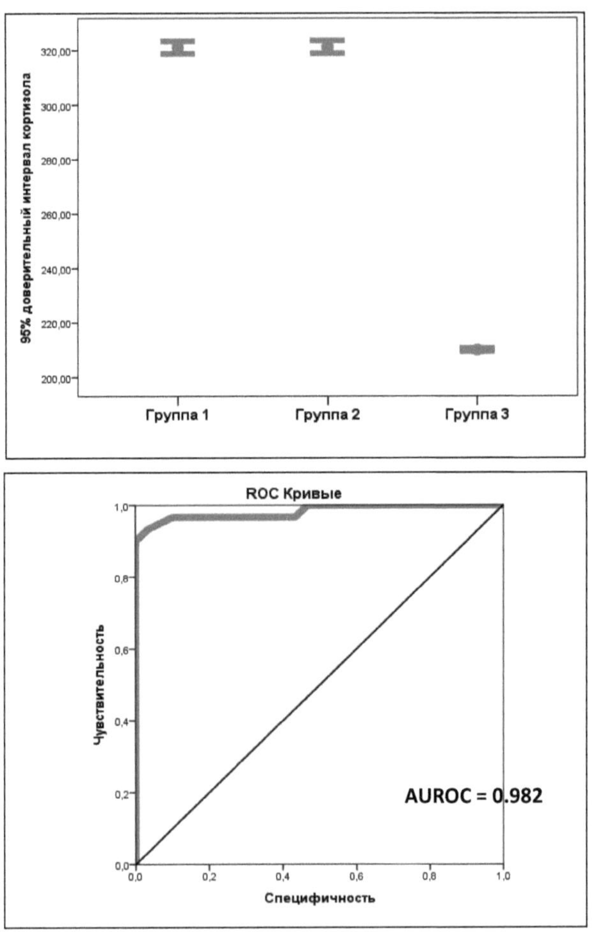

Figure 35. 95% confidence intervals of cortisol levels in the blood of women in the Russian population and ROC curves the predictive value of the test

(pink colour indicates the reference value area)

Finally, cortisol levels as a marker of reproductive impairment, as Figure 35 shows, were highly significant in the Russian population of women, as defined by an AUROC value of 0.982 in the zone of values approximately below 215 nmol/l.

It is also necessary to emphasise the fact that all established markers of reproductive health disorders did not exceed the reference values, although they were, as a rule, at their upper or lower limits.

4.1.3 Ranges of prognostically important values of indicators hormonal status in a risk group of Russian women

The objective of this research section was to clarify the ranges of prognostically important values of markers of risk group 3 in the population of Russian women. For this purpose, the borderline values of 95% confidence intervals (95% CI) of all the markers obtained were compared by study group, taking into account their standard deviations. The results of this study are presented in Table 15.

When prognostically significant values in group 3 exceeded the 95% confidence intervals in the other groups, the lower limits of these intervals for prognostically significant indicators and the upper limits for the same indicators in the other two groups were compared, with the maximum value in the comparison groups being taken as the limit of the prognostically significant range.

In those cases when prognostically significant values in group 3 exceeded 95% confidence intervals in other groups, the upper limits of these intervals for prognostically significant indicators and the lower limits for the same indicators in the other two groups were used for comparison, and the minimum value among the values in the comparison groups was taken as the boundary of the prognostically significant range.

Table 15. Borderline values and prognostic

significant values for hormone levels in women

of the Russian population in the study groups

Informative indicators	**Upper/ lower boundary for groups 1**	**Upper/ lower boundary for groups 2**	**Upper/ lower boundary for groups of 3**	**Prognostically meaningful range values in group 3**
Luteinising hormone (IU/L)	max 5,1	max 5,0	min 5,1	> 5.1 ME/l
Prolactin (mME/ml)	max 134,2	max 136,0	min 300,1	> 136 mMU/ml
Estradiol (pmol/l)	max 236,0	max 237	min 297,2	> 237 pmol/l
Progesterone (nmol/l)	max 26,5	max 26,0	min 53,8	> 26.5 nmol/l
Thyroid hormone (mME/l)	max 1,6	max 1,0	min 1,6	> 1.6 mIU/l
Total thyroxine (nmol/l)	max 86,3	max 86,5	min 123,4	> 86.5 nmol/l
Cortisol (nmol/l)	min 291	min 291	max 212,3	< 291 nmol/l

Note: grey indicates borderline prognostically significant value

As follows from the table, the performance of this fragment of studies made it possible to establish prognostically significant values that allow us to establish the boundary value of the indicator, beyond which it can be considered a sign (marker) of reproductive dysfunction, either upward or downward (depending on the direction of the prognostically significant deviation). In cases where the values of the indicator were within the prognostically significant range, especially in the absence of obstetric history, a woman could be assigned to the appropriate risk group.

4.2 Hormonal status and risk groups for disorders Reproductive health of women in the Tajik population

4.2.1 Sex hormones and risk groups for disorders Reproductive function in Tajik women

Hormonal status in the population of Tajik women was analysed according to the scheme similar to that outlined in Section 4.1. Table 16 and Figure 36 present the results of such analyses on the content of sex hormones in the blood of women of different groups.

Table 16.

Sex hormone levels in women Tajik population in the study groups

Informative indicators	Median indicator [minimum, maximum]			p_1 p_2 p_3
	Group 5	Group 6	Group 7	
FSH (IU/L)	4,0 [1,6; 7,9]	3,8 [1,9; 5,3]	4,0 [0,4; 8,5]	0,313 0,731 0,706
LH (IU/L)	5,1 [1,4; 8,9]	4,2 [2,8; 5,6]	5,1 [3,9; 7,9]	0,010 <0,001 0,922
Prolactin (mME/ml)	210,0 [138,0; 213,5]	124,4 [121,0; 141,0]	210,1 [205,5; 213,9]	<0,001 <0,001 0,737
Estradiol (pmol/l)	249,1 [238,6; 253,4]	231,6 [220,3; 241,5]	250,0 [245,8; 253,0]	<0,001 <0,001 0,413
Progesterone (nmol/l)	35,6 [29,1; 38,0]	21,2 [17,9; 30,0]	35,4 [29,4; 37,2]	<0,001 <0,001 0,588
17-OP (nmol/l)	3,0 [1,4; 4,8]	3,4 [1,6; 5,0]	3,0 [0,7; 4,9]	0,694 0,654 0,465
Testosterone (nmol/l)	1,6 [0,1; 4,1]	2,2 [1,1; 4,0]	2,0 [0,1; 5,2]	0,001 0,290 0,253
DHEAc (nmol/l)	4,4 [2,2; 6,8]	5,6 [3,7; 7,9]	3,9 [2,4; 8,9]	0,001 <0,001 0,431

Note: p_1 - probability of differences between groups 5 and 6; p_2 - probability of differences between groups 6 and 7; p_3 - probability of differences between groups 5 and 7; grey indicates the significance of differences ($p<0.05$) according to the Mann-Whitney test.

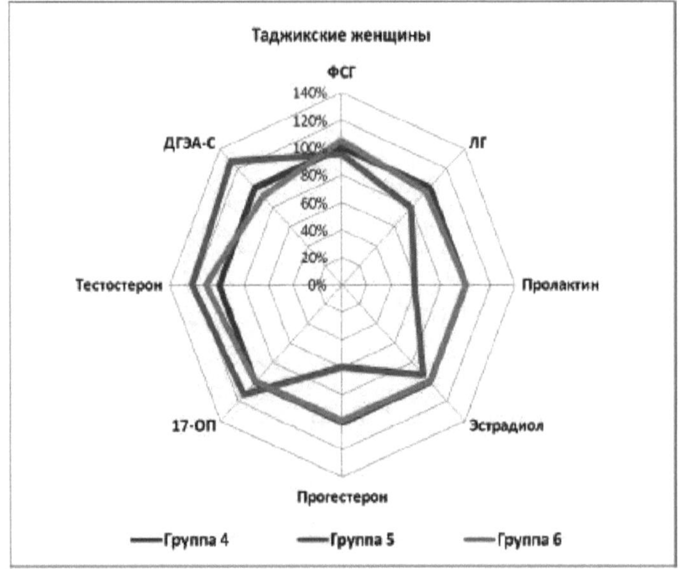

Figure 36. Percentages of variation in sex hormone levels in Tajik women with reproductive disorders from those of healthy women

(* - differences between the values of indicators are statistically reliable)

In the category of Tajik women, reliable deviations from the control (indicators in women with preserved reproductive health) are of a different nature than in the Russian population, although they also affect only one of the risk groups - group 6. In this group, there is a significant drop in the blood content of all sex hormones, except for androgens, the level of which is increasing. In terms of androgens, there is another difference in the respective groups of different populations: in the Russian women's population, a drop in testosterone levels is indicative, while in the Tajik women's population, an increase in dihydroepiandrosterone levels is indicative.

Next, we tested all of the above hormones, except for follicle-stimulating hormone and 17-OH progesterone, which showed no significant intergroup differences, as markers of hormonal disorders in the respective risk groups. For this purpose, the 95% confidence intervals of each of the informative hormones were determined to determine the ranges of their values in which they appear as markers, and then the degree of their prognostic significance was established by constructing ROC curves and calculating AUROC, as shown in Figures 37-42.

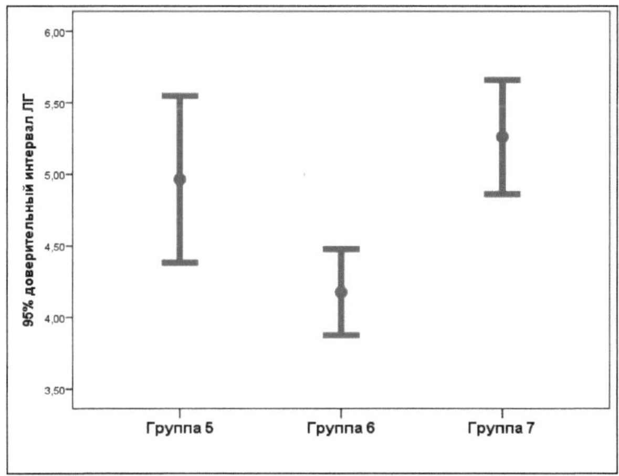

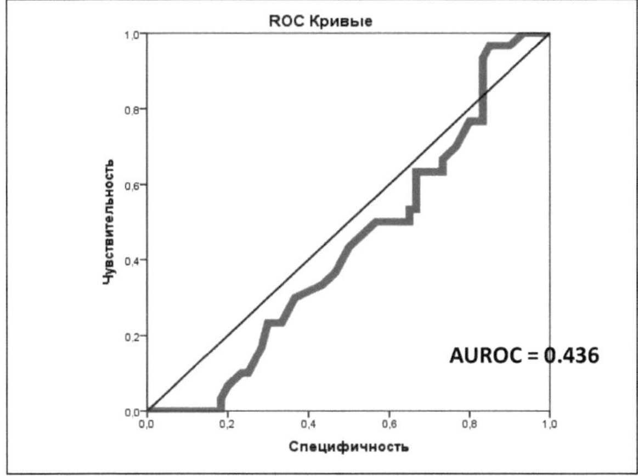

Figure 37. 95% confidence intervals for luteinising lutein levels of hormone in the blood of Tajik women of the study groups and ROC curve of the predictive value of the test
(green colour indicates the reference value area)

As can be seen from the graph in Figure 37, in the population of Tajik women, despite the reliability of the differences in group levels of luteinising hormone noted in Table 7, the latter was not confirmed at the level of their prognostic significance as a marker of reproductive health disorders, since the 95% confidence intervals of luteinising hormone in different groups partially overlapped with each other, and the AUROC was only 0.436.

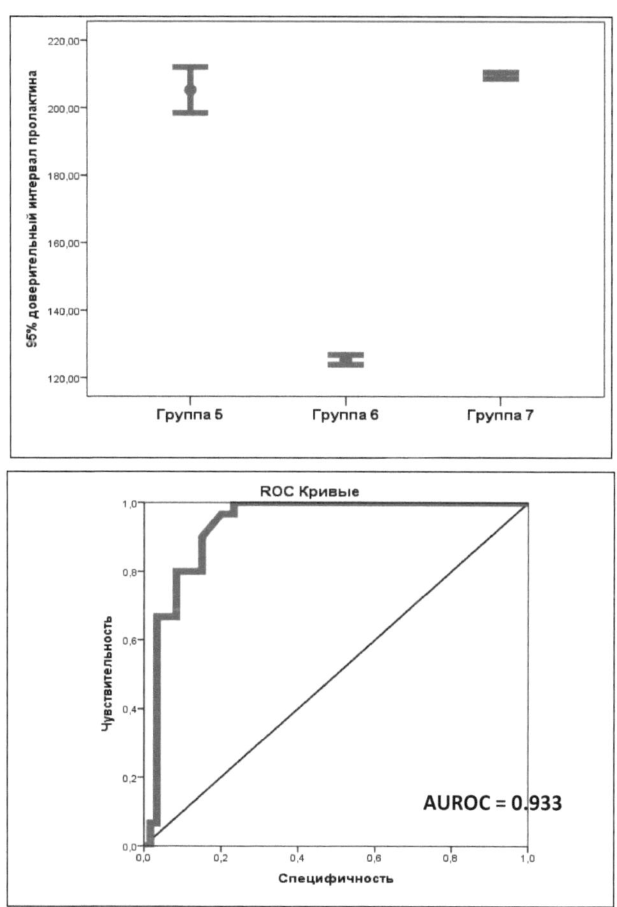

Figure 38. 95% confidence intervals of prolactin levels in the blood of Tajik women of the study groups and ROC curve of the predictive value of the test
(green colour indicates the reference value area)

Figure 38 clearly shows that the level of another pituitary hormone, prolactin, is a fairly reliable prognostic indicator of whether women in the Tajik population are at risk of reproductive disorders (group 6). In the latter case, the prognostically significant prolactin values fell below 140 mIU/ml, and the AUROC value indicated a very high prognostic value of the test, as it was equal to 0.933.

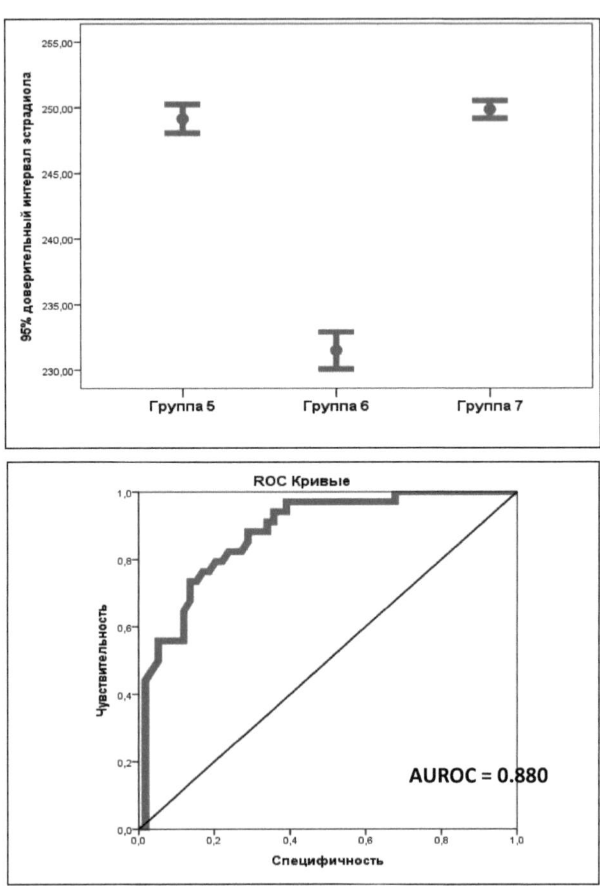

Figure 39. 95% confidence intervals of estradiol levels in the blood of Tajik women of the study groups and ROC curve of the predictive value of the test

(green colour indicates the reference value area)

Ovarian hormones, particularly oestradiol (Figure 39), were also found to have high predictive value, as presented in Figure 39. Like other sex hormones, the 95% confidence interval for oestradiol was significantly lower in the group of 6 Tajik women (<240 pmol/l). The prognostic significance of these abnormalities was very high because the area under the ROC curve (AUROC) was 0.880.

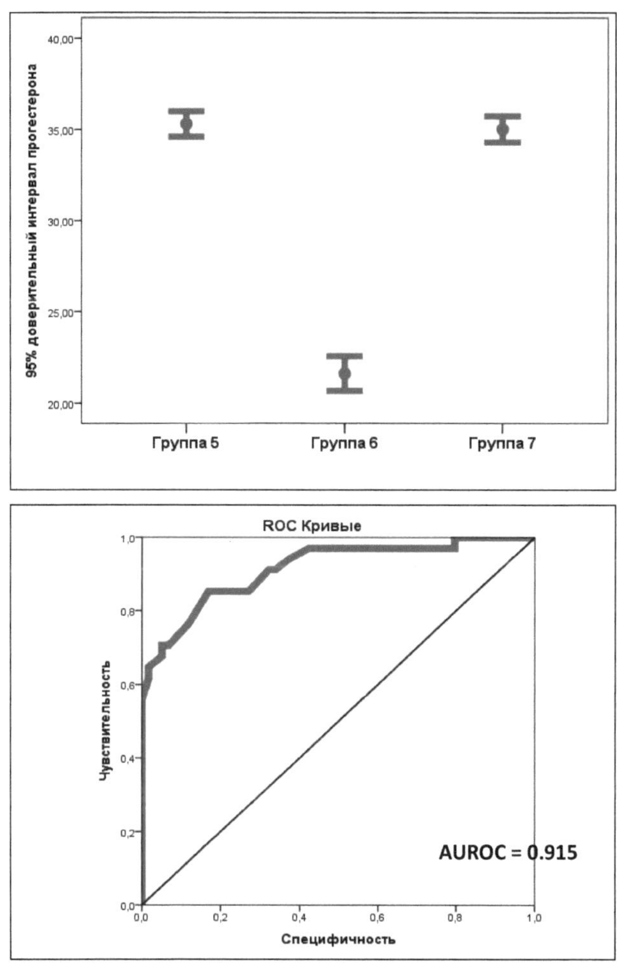

Figure 40. 95% confidence intervals of progesterone levels in the blood of Tajik women in the study groups and ROC curve of the predictive value of the test
(green colour indicates the reference value area)

Another important ovarian hormone, progesterone, was also highly prognostic with an AUROC of 0.915, as shown in Figure 40. In the Tajik population, a progesterone level below 30 nmol/L indicated that the woman belonged to risk group 6.

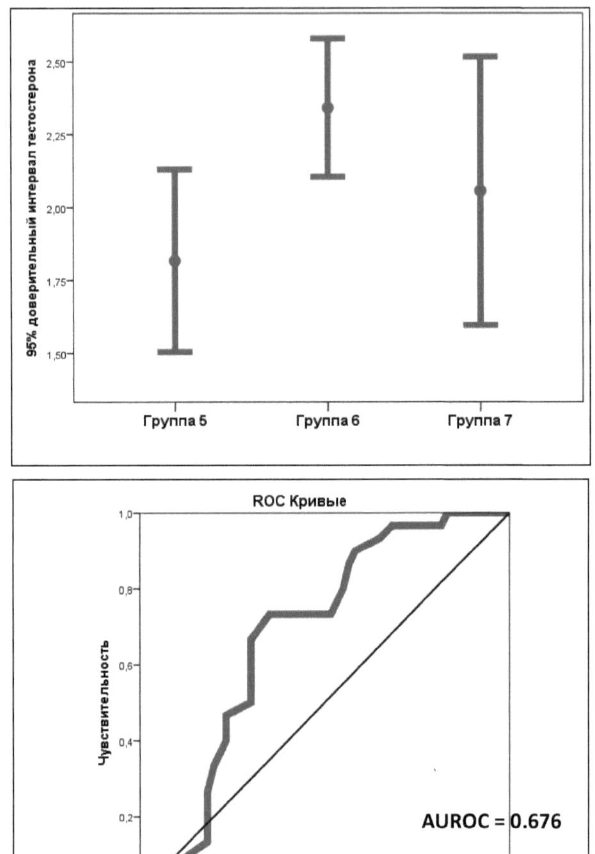

Figure 41. 95% confidence intervals of testosterone levels in the blood of Tajik women of the study groups and ROC curve of the predictive value of the test

(green colour indicates the reference value area)

Figure 41 shows the results of assessing the prognostic role of testosterone, a male sex hormone produced in the female body by the ovaries and adrenal glands. This hormone can hardly claim to be a marker of reproductive disorders, since in Tajik women the AUROC value showed moderate prognostic significance and was equal to 0.676.

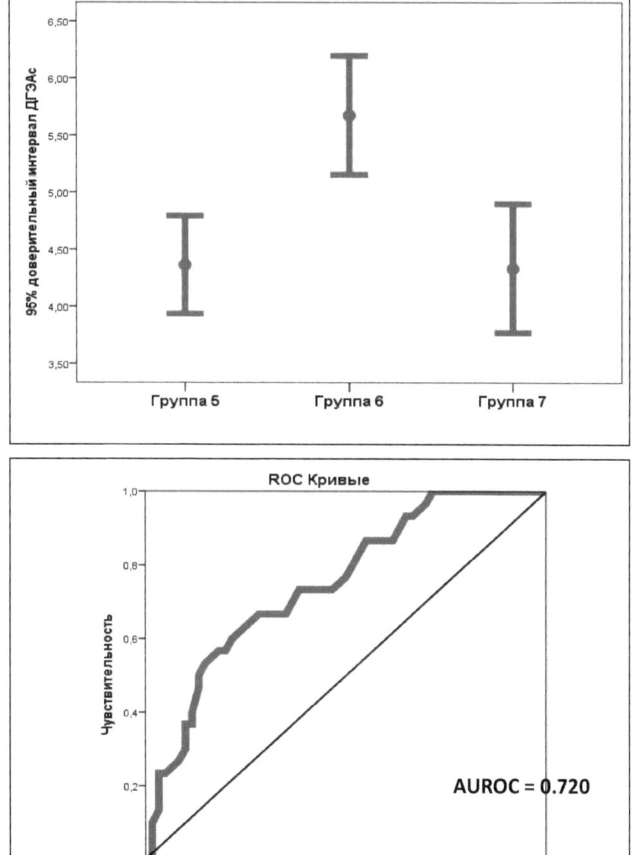

Figure 42. 95% confidence intervals of lihydroepialdosterone sulphate levels in the blood of Tajik women of the study groups and ROC curve of the predictive value of the test
(green colour indicates the reference value area)

The testosterone metabolite dihydroepiandrosterone, as shown in Figure 42, was consistent with that of testosterone in its prognostic significance, which was moderate in the Tajik population (AUROC = 0.720).

Thus, the studies conducted in this section have confirmed that the pathogenesis of reproductive disorders in women of the Tajik population may be based on a decrease in the level of female sex hormones in the blood and an increase in androgens, while the content of prolactin, oestradiol and progesterone in the blood can be used as markers of a woman's belonging to a risk group with a history of reproductive health disorders.

4.2.2 Thyroid and adrenal hormones and groups risk of women's reproductive health problems Tajik population

This section of research is devoted to the study of the role of thyroid and adrenal hormones in the development of reproductive pathology from the perspective of population-cluster approach at the prenosological stage.

The results of this study in a population of Tajik women divided into groups (clusters) based on obstetric history are presented in Table 17 and Figure 43. The objects of the study in this case were blood levels of the following hormones: thyroid hormone, total triiodothyronine (T3), total thyroxine (T4), cortisol, and autoantibodies to thyroglobulin and thyroperoxidase.

As follows from the presented data, the level of thyroid hormones, autoantibodies to thyroid components, cortisol has a pronounced peculiarity in a part of women with reproductive disorders belonging to the Tajik population.

Table 17. Hormonal status in women Tajik population by study group

Informative indicators	Median indicator [minimum, maximum]			p_1 p_2 p_3
	Group 5	Group 6	Group 7	
Thyroid hormone (mME/l)	1,6 [0,7; 2,5]	0,6 [0,1; 1,9]	1,7 [0,1; 3,1]	<0,001 <0,001 0,320
Total T3 (nmol/l)	2,1 [0,1; 3,4]	1,5 [0,5; 2,9]	2,1 [0,2; 3,5]	0,028 0,031 0,844
Total T4 (nmol/ml)	100,1 [97,6; 102,6]	80,1 [78,3; 83,5]	100,0 [97,0; 120,0]	<0,001 <0,001 0,838
Autoantibodies to thyroglobulin (IU/ml)	2,7 [2,0; 4,0]	4,2 [4,1; 4,25]	2,7 [2,6; 2,9]	<0,001 <0,001 0,647
Autoantibodies to thyroperoxidase (IU/ml)	11,8 [10,8; 12,8]	22,7 [22,3; 23,5]	12,0 [11,0; 40,1]	<0,001 <0,001 0,384
Cortisol (nmol/l)	250,6 [246,8; 331,0]	340,0 [336,8; 350,0]	250,6 [248,7; 253,6]	<0,001 <0,001 0,544

Note: p_1 - probability of differences in groups 1 and 2; p_2 - probability of differences in groups 2 and 3; p_3 - probability of differences in data in groups 1 and 3; grey indicates the significance of differences ($p<0.05$) by the Mann-Whitney test

For example, women in the Tajik population belonging to group 6 in terms of reproductive disorders, along with reduced levels of sex hormones in the blood, have decreased levels of thyroid hormones. The degree of such a decrease was significant in all cases, which was quite understandable from the point of view of the severity of the autoimmune component registered ro in these studies. The fact is that in women of group 6 parall lely there was a rather significant increase in the blood content of autoantibodies to thyroid components - thyroglobulin and thyroo peroxidase.

As for the adrenal hormone cortisol, its content in the blood of women in the Tajik population was 1.5 times higher in the case of women belonging to the risk group for reproductive disorders.

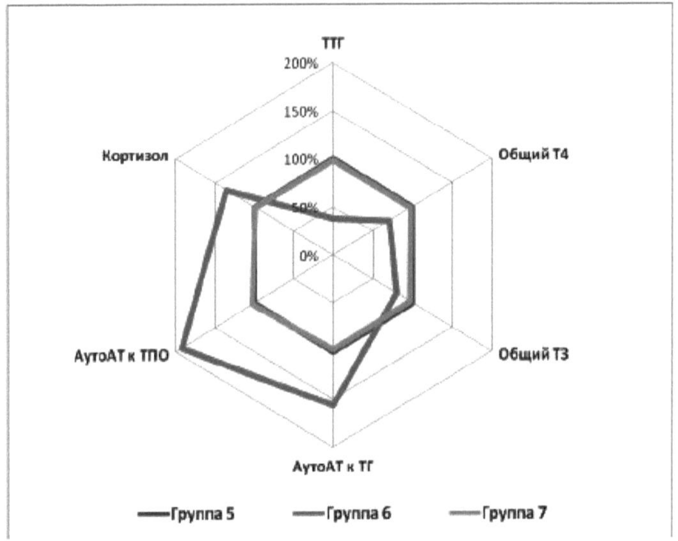

Figure 43. Percentages of deviation of hormonal status indicators
Women with reproductive disorders in the Tajik population from healthy women

(* - differences between the values of indicators are statistically reliable)

To address the question of what changes in thyroid and adrenal functions may serve as markers of reproductive disorders in these groups, as well as in other cases, 95% confidence intervals were determined and a ROC curve was constructed with calculation of the AUROC value. The data of such studies are presented in Figures 44-49.

Figure 44 shows the 95% confidence intervals and ROC curve for thyroid hormone levels in different groups of women in the Tajik population. It was found that the 95% confidence interval for thyroid hormone levels differed downward in Group 6, in which reproductive disorders were identified in the analysis of obstetric history, but the degree of difference was moderate, as the AUROC was 0.720, with all deviations occurring within the reference values of the indicator, as in other cases.

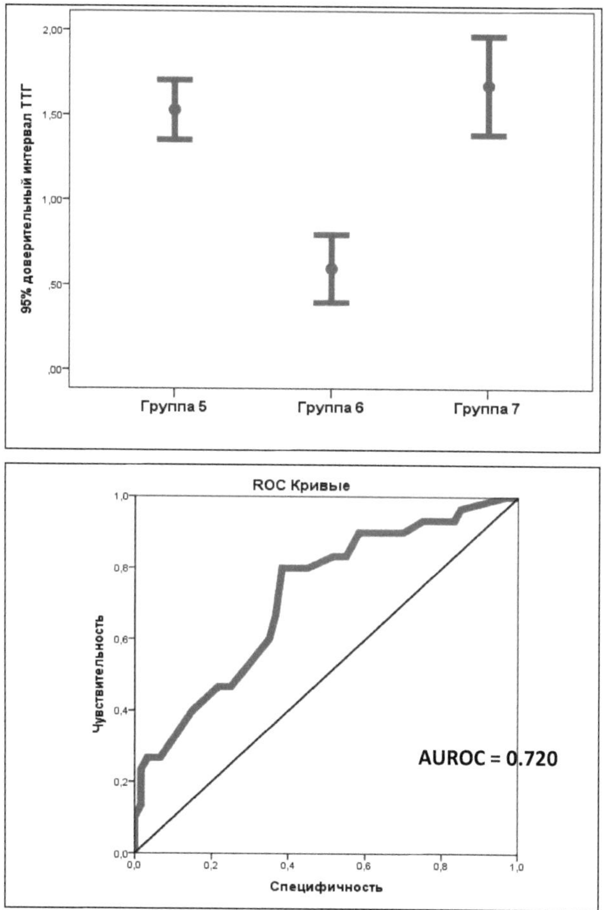

Figure 44. 95% confidence intervals of thyroid hormone levels in the blood of Tajik women of the study groups and the ROC curve of the predictive value of the test

(green colour indicates the reference value area)

As Figure 45 shows, the content of total triiodothyronine in the blood can hardly claim to be a marker of possible reproductive disorders, since in the population of Tajik women this indicator demonstrated only low prognostic significance (AUROC = 0.562).

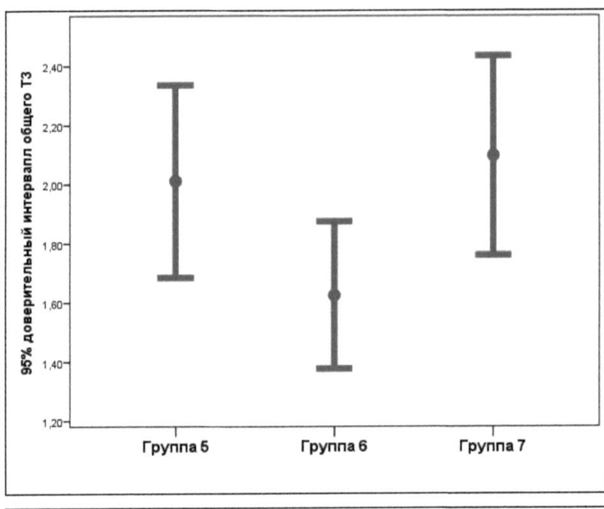

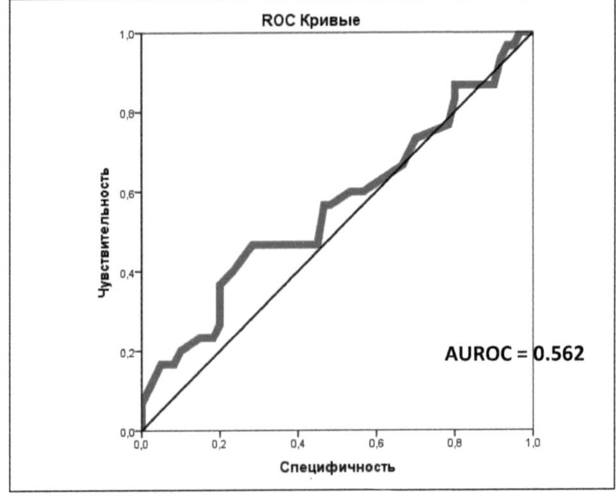

Figure 45. 95% confidence intervals of total triiodothyronine levels
in the blood of Tajik women of the study groups and the ROC curve of the predictive value of the test
(green colour indicates the reference value area)

Similar results were obtained for the level of total thyroxine in the blood (Figure 46), as the determination of intergroup differences for this thyroid hormone showed that in Tajik women this indicator had a relative diagnostic value in group 6, but was only moderately significant (AUROC=0.759).

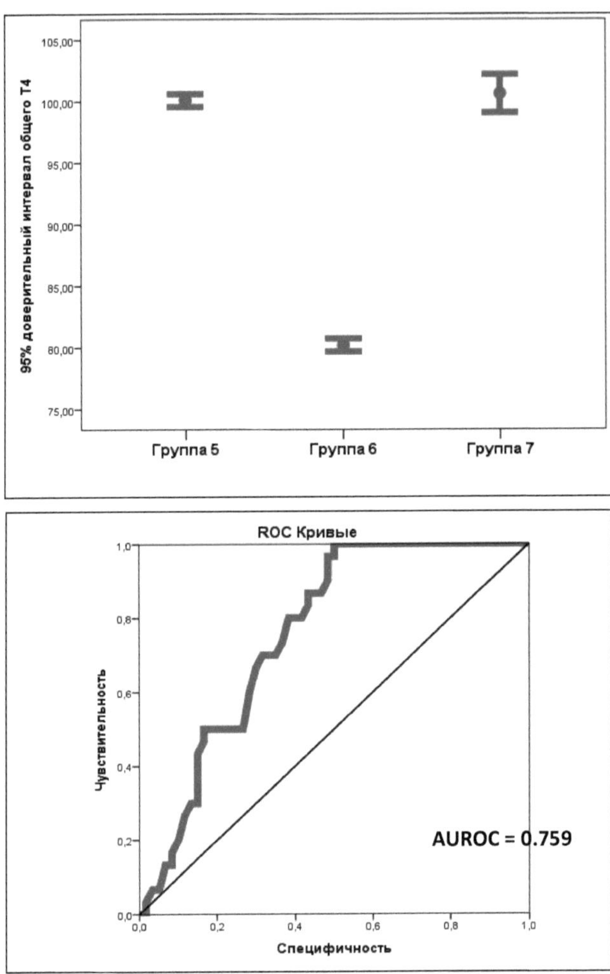

Figure 46. 95% confidence intervals of total thyroxine levels in the blood of Tajik women of the study groups and the ROC curve of the predictive value of the test

(green colour indicates the reference value area)

Quite unambiguous were such indicators as levels of autoan titel to thyroid components, as it is presented according to the results of statistical processing in Figures 47 and 48.

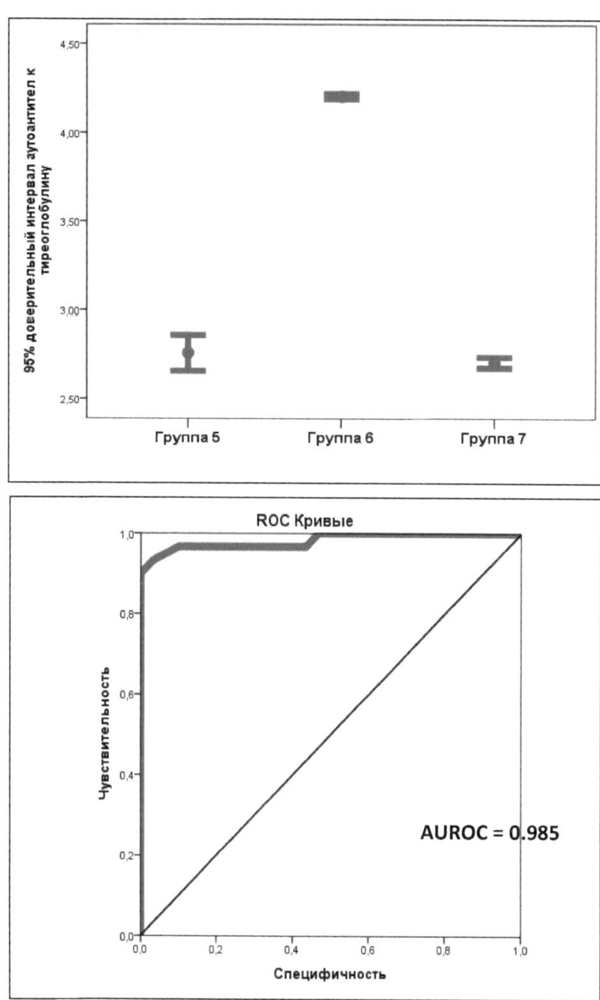

Figure 47. 95% confidence intervals of thyroglobulin autoantibody levels in the blood of Tajik women of the study groups and ROC-curve of the predictive value of the test
(green colour indicates the reference value area)

In women of the Tajik population, the level of autoantibodies to thyroid proteins was significantly elevated in one of the risk groups - group 6 (thyroglobulin>3.5 IU/ml, thyroperoxidase >18 IU/ml). This elevation showed, judging by AUROC values (0.985-1.0), a very high prognostic significance approaching absolute.

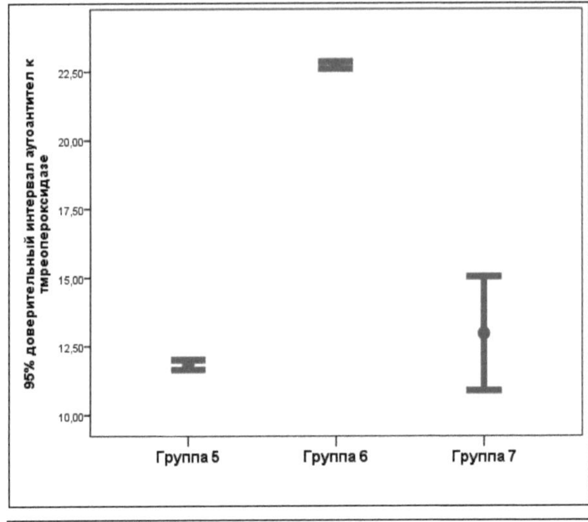

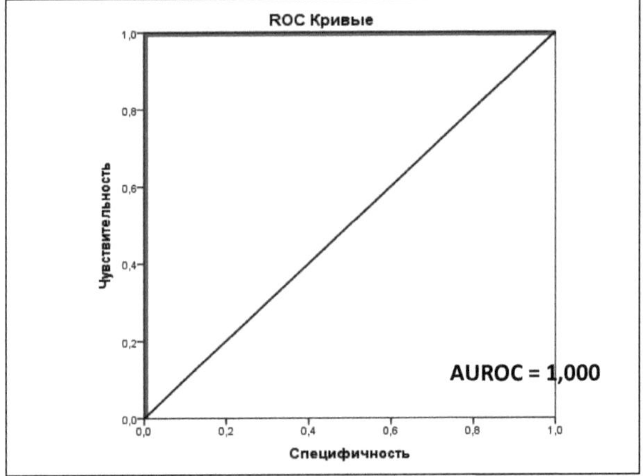

Figure 48. 95% confidence intervals of thyroperoxidase autoantibody levels in the blood of Tajik women of the study groups and ROC curve of the predictive value of the test
(green colour indicates the reference value area)

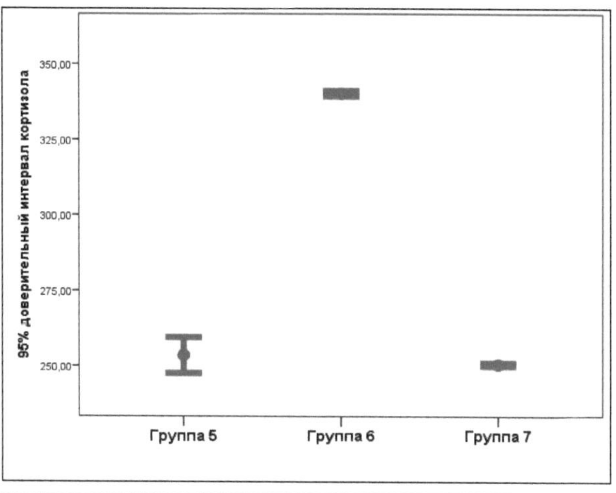

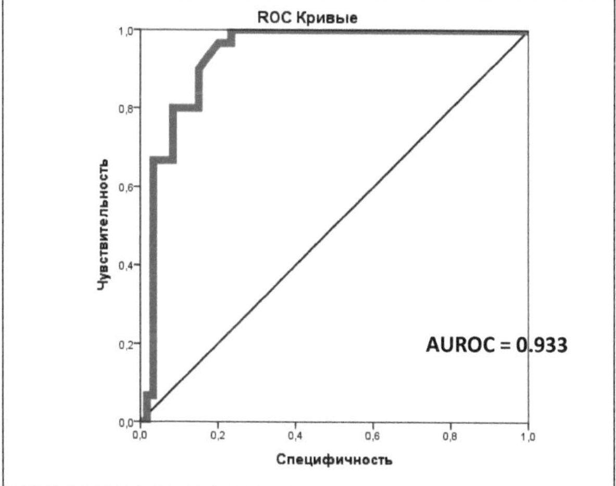

Figure 49. 95% confidence intervals of cortisol levels in the blood of Tajik women of the study groups and ROC-curve of the predictive value of the test
(green colour indicates the reference value area)

Finally, the cortisol level as a marker of reproductive health impairment (this follows from Figure 49), was highly significant. As in the Russian population, in Tajik women its prognostic significance was determined by the AUROC value of 0.933 in the zone of values above 330 nmol/l.

4.2.3 Ranges of prognostically important values of indicators Hormonal status in a risk group of Tajik women

The objective of this section of the study was to clarify the ranges of prognostically important values of markers of risk group 6 in the population of Tajik women. As in the case of the Russian population, we compared the borderline values of 95% confidence intervals of all obtained markers by study group, taking into account their standard deviations. The results of this study are presented in Table 18.

Table 18. Borderline values and prognostic significant values for hormone levels in women Tajik population in the study groups

Informative indicators	**Upper/ lower boundar y for groups of 5**	**Upper/ lower boundar y for groups of 6**	**Upper/ lower boundar y for groups of 7**	**Prognostic ally significant range values in group 6**
Prolactin (mME/ml)	min 207	max 129	min 205	< 205 mMU/ml
Estradiol (pmol/l)	min 247	max 236	min 245	< 245 pmol/l
Progesterone (nmol/l)	min 33,4	max 26,0	min 32,5	> 32.5 nmol/l
Autoantibodies to thyroglobulin (IU/ml)	max 2,8	min 4,2	max 2,9	> 2.9 mIU/l
Autoantibodies to thyro-peroxidase (IU/ml)	max 12,8	min 22,5	min 15,7	> 15.7 nmol/l

Cortisol (nmol/l)	max 253	min 337	max 254	> 254 nmol/l

Note: grey indicates borderline prognostically significant value

As follows from the table, the implementation of this fragment of research allowed us to establish prognostically significant values, which allow us to establish those borderline values of indicators, beyond which (depending on the direction of prognostically significant deviation) they can be considered as signs (markers) of reproductive disorders in the population of Tajik women. The presence of such shifts in a woman, not exceeding the reference values, can serve as a sign of her reproductive health disorders at the preclinical stage.

Summary to chapter 4

1. In the population of Russian women with a history of pregnancy failure, premature births and stillborn children, a risk group characterised by abnormalities of hormonal status within the reference values for luteinising hormone, prolactin, oestradiol, progesterone, thyroid hormone, total thyroxine, and cortisol is identified, which does not include all women with reproductive disorders. .
2. In the population of Tajik women with impaired reproductive function, there is a contingent with shifts in hormonal status within the reference range of prolactin, estradiol, progesterone, high levels of autoantibodies to thyrogl bulin and thyro peroxidase, and cortisol, which does not cover all women with reproductive pathology.
3. Markers of reproductive health disorders among indicators of hormonal status and ranges of informative values of these

markers in the studied populations of Russian and Tajik women are presented in Table 19:

Table 19. Markers of hormonal shifts associated with with reproductive health problems

Studied populations	Marker is an indicator hormonal status	Value range marker
Russian population women, group 3	Luteinising hormone	> 5.1 ME/l
	Prolactin	> 136 mMU/ml
	Estradiol	> 237 pmol/l
	Progesterone	> 26.5 nmol/l
	Thyroid hormone	> 1.6 mIU/l
	Total thyroxine	> 86.5 nmol/l
	Cortisol	< 291 nmol/l
Tajik Women's Population, group 6	Prolactin	< 205 mMU/ml
	Estradiol	< 245 pmol/l
	Progesterone	> 32.5 nmol/l
	Autoantibodies to thyroglobulin	> 2.9 mIU/l
	Autoantibodies to thyroperoxidase	> 15.7 nmol/l
	Cortisol	> 254 nmol/l

CHAPTER 5. IMMUNE STATUS, ANTIPHOSPHOLIPID REACTIONS AND RISK GROUPS FOR REPRODUCTIVE HEALTH DISORDERS IN WOMEN

5.1 Immune status and risk groups for disorders Reproductive health of women in the Russian population

The objective of this section of the research was to identify markers of risk of reproductive health disorders among the indicators characterising the immune status of women in the Russian population. Such indicators included phenotypic characteristics of blood lymphocytes, levels of immunoglobulins in blood serum, and the content of autoantibodies in blood serum to hemostasis components characterising the state of antiphospholipid reactions.

5.1.1 Phenotypic characterisation of lymphocytes and groups at risk of reproductive health problems of women in the Russian population

Among all the variety of abnormalities associated with reproductive health disorders, a certain role belongs to changes in immune status, in particular, in the blood content of lymphocytes of different phenotypes.

The results of the study of phenotypic characteristics in the population of Russian women belonging to different reproductive health groups in the form of direct immunogram data are presented in Table 20 and in the form of the percentage of deviations of the indicators of the 2 risk groups from those in the group of women with preserved reproductive function - in Figure 50.

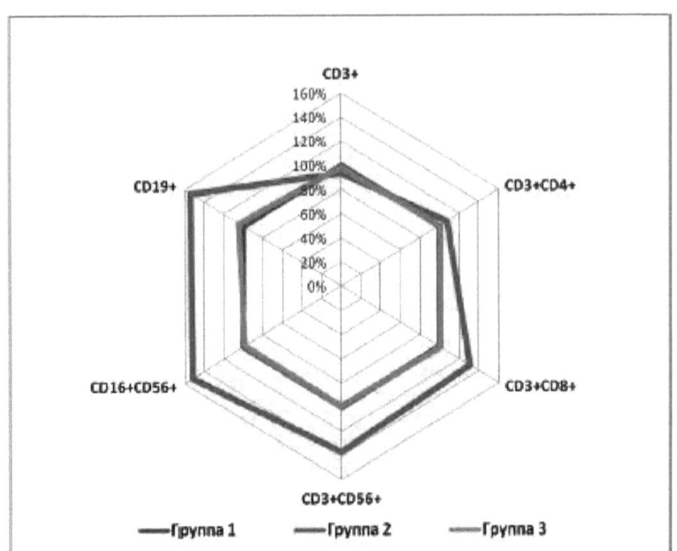

Figure 50. Percentages of variation in the number of lymphocytes of different phenotypes in the blood of Russian women with reproductive disorders from those with reproductive disorders in healthy women
(* - differences between the values of indicators are statistically reliable)

As the data obtained show, the nature of changes in immunophenotypic indicators using the population cluster approach does not fully correspond to those in the assessment of hormonal status, since the latter affected another group with reproductive health disorders in Russian women - group 2, while the main deviations in hormonal status were registered, as has already been noted, in group 3. The figure clearly shows that despite the fact that almost every analysed immunophenotypic indicator in group 2 gave reliable deviations from the indicators of healthy women, the degree of such deviations was different. The greatest upward shifts were observed in the cells with potential cytotoxic activity - cytotoxic T-lymphocytes (CD3+CD8+), natural killer cells (CD16+CD56+), EKT (CD3+CD56+). A significant increase in the number of B-lymphocytes (CD19+) was also observed.

Table 20. Percentage of lymphocytes of different phenotypes in the blood of women of the Russian population in the study groups

Informative indicators	Median indicator [minimum, maximum]			p_1 p_2 p_3
	Group 1	Group 2	Group 3	
1	2	3	4	5
T-lymphocytes are. CD3+	71,4 [67,4; 74,5]	66,9 [64,3; 71,4]	71,3 [66,2; 74,5]	<0,001 <0,001 0,294
T-helper cells CD3+CD4+	34,7 [32,2; 37,6]	37,3 [35,7; 40,2]	35,0 [31,0; 37,6]	<0,001 <0,001 0,952
Cytotoxic T-lymphocytes - CD3+CD8+	18,4 [16,1; 19,6]	24,2 [21,5; 28,3]	18,6 [16,1; 20,1]	<0,001 <0,001 0,405
EKT - CD3+CD56+	3,6 [2,1; 4,2]	5,0 [3,7; 7,0]	3,6 [2,5; 4,1]	<0,001 <0,001 0,596
1	2	3	4	5
Natural killers - CD16+CD56+	11,8 [10,1; 14,5]	17,9 [15,9; 20,4]	11,7 [10,0; 13,8]	<0,001 <0,001 0,510
B-lymphocytes - CD19+	6,2 [4,5; 9,3]	10,4 [5,6; 13,6]	6,9 [4,8; 9,3]	<0,001 <0,001 0,388

Note: p_1 - probability of data differences in groups 1 and 2; p_2 - probability of data differences in groups 2 and 3; p_3 - probability of data differences in groups 1 and 3; grey shows significance of differences ($p<0.05$) by Mann-Whitney test

The obtained data created a prerequisite for creating a system of immuno phenotypic markers of reproductive health disorders in women in group 2 of the Russian population by analysing all tested indicators on the basis of their 95% confidence intervals and their corresponding ROC curves (Figures 51-56).

Figure 51 shows the results of determining the 95% confidence intervals of the relative number of T-lymphocytes in the blood by individual groups in the population of Russian women. This indicator was reduced only in one of the groups with reproductive health disorders - group 2. At the same time, the prognostic significance of this test was, although close to high values, still moderate, as AUROC = 0.766. In other words, in the presence of other markers with a high level of prognostic significance, this indicator can be neglected.

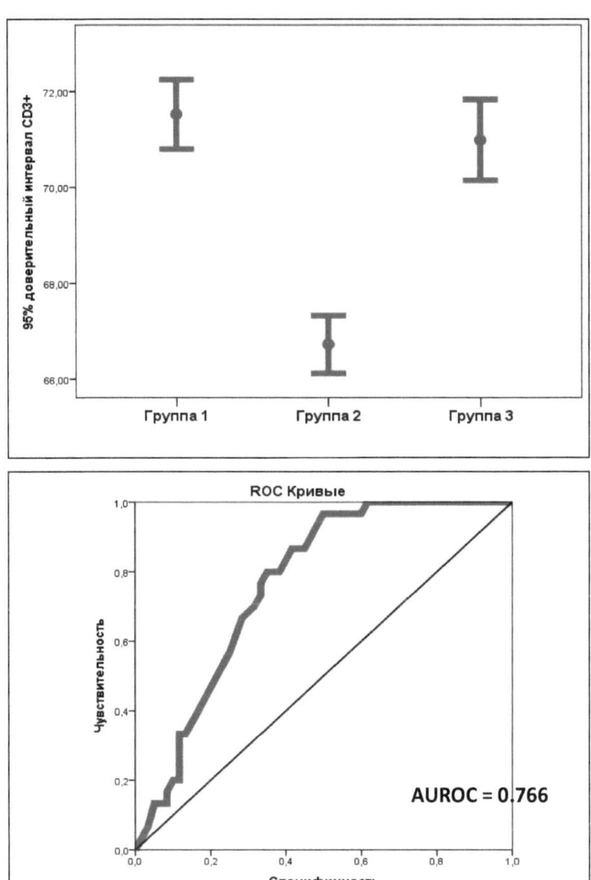

Figure 51. 95% confidence intervals of T-lymphocyte counts in the blood of Russian women of the study groups and ROC curve the predictive value of the test
(green colour indicates the reference value area)

Figure 52 shows the 95% confidence limits for one of the main subpopulations of T-lymphocytes - T-helper cells (CD3+CD4+). When the relative number of these cells was approximately higher than 36% in group 2 of Russian women, the prognostic significance of the test was high, as the AUROC value was 0.890.

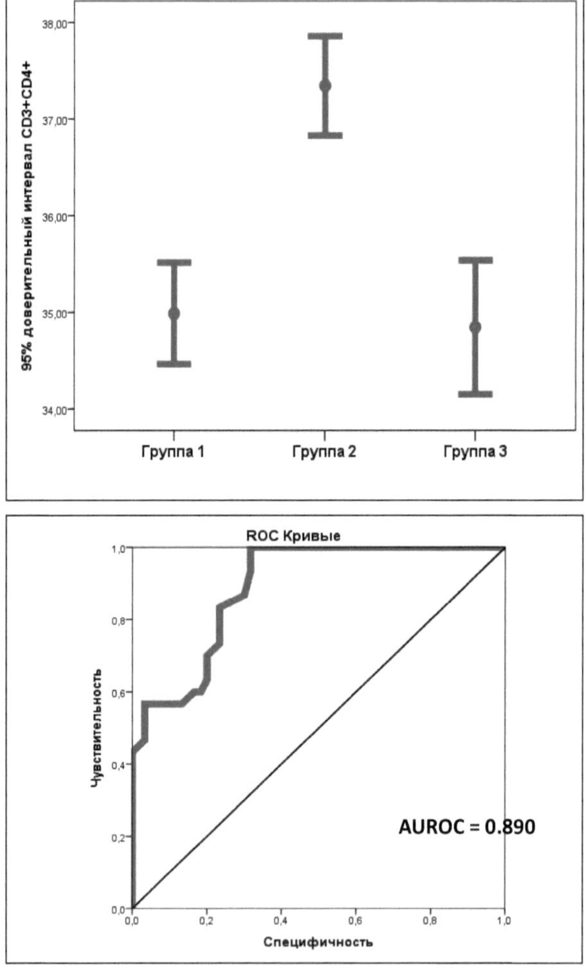

Figure 52. 95% confidence intervals of the number of T-helper cells

in the blood of Russian women of the study groups and ROC curve
the predictive value of the test
(green colour indicates the reference value area)

The relative number of cytotoxic T lymphocytes (CD3+CD8+) was also highly prognostically significant (AUROC = 1.0), as shown in Figure 53. In group 2 of the Russian population, the number of CTLs had such significance with values approximately above 21%.

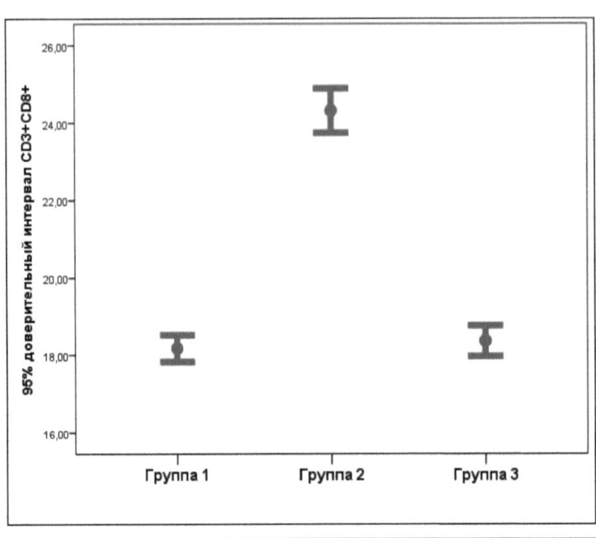

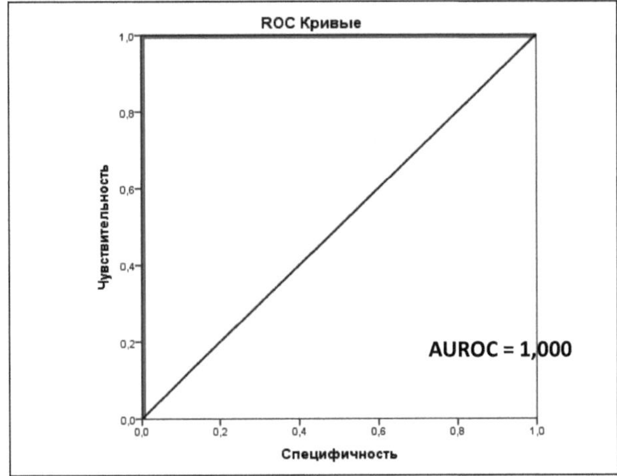

Figure 53. 95% confidence intervals of the number of cytotoxic T-lymphocytes in the blood of Russian women of the studied groups and ROC curves of the predictive value of the test
(green colour indicates the reference value area)

High prognostic significance (AUROC=0.967) was also demonstrated by the percentage of ECT among blood lymphocytes

(Figure 54). In the Russian population, this indicator had marker signs when its value increased approximately above 4.3%.

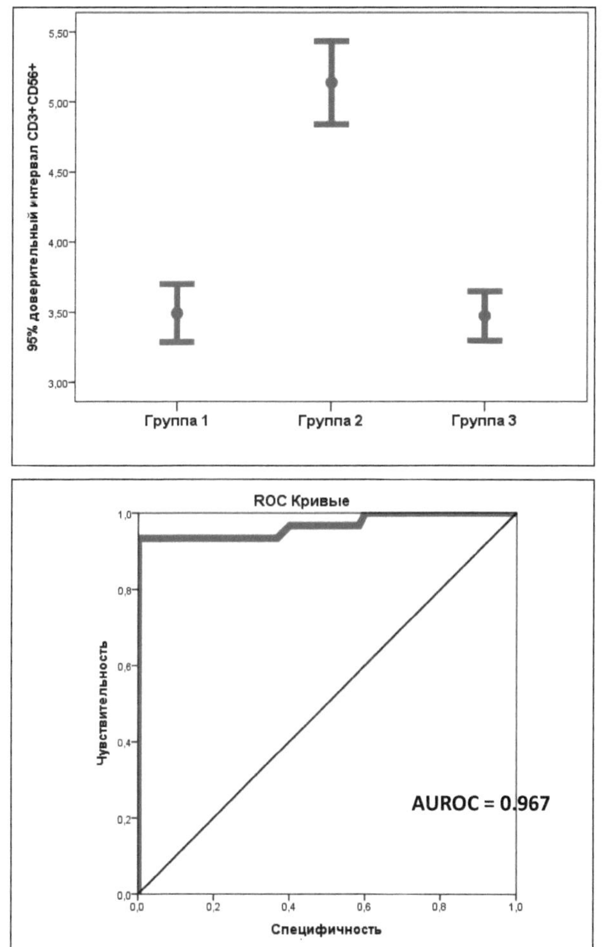

Figure 54. 95% confidence intervals of the number of ECTs in blood Russian women in the study groups and ROC curve the predictive value of the test

(green colour indicates the reference value area)

The relative number of natural killer cells (Figure 55) turned out to be the most important prognostic sign when performing phenotyping of blood lymphocytes, since the AUROC value, which is a quantitative criterion of such significance, was close to absolute and was 1.0. The percentage of ECs among blood lymphocytes was approximately higher than 15% in group 2 of the Russian population.

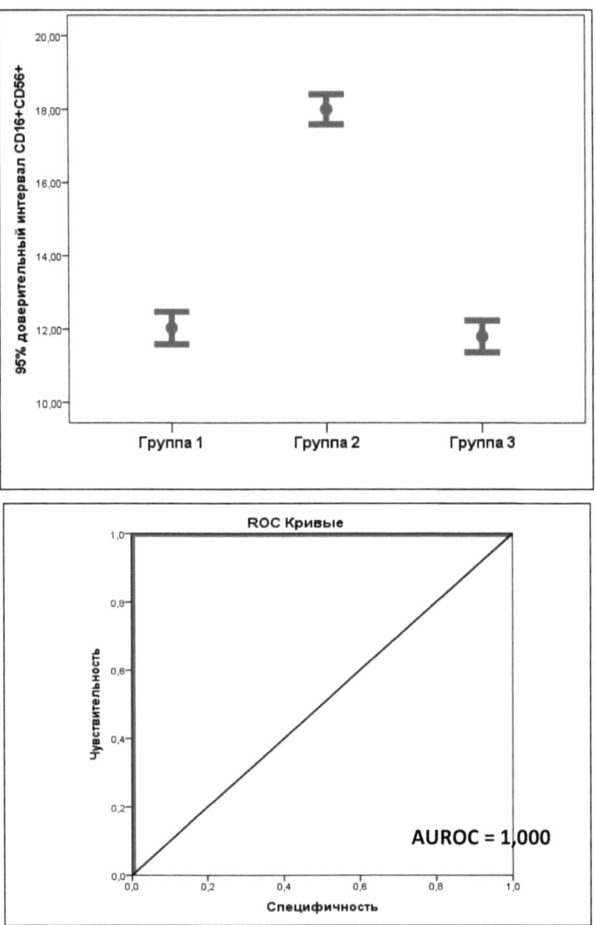

Figure 55. 95% confidence intervals of the number of natural killer cells in the blood of Russian women of the study groups and ROC curve the predictive value of the test

(green colour indicates the reference value area)

The content of B-lymphocytes in the blood of women with reproductive disorders can also claim to be a marker of such disorders (Figure 56). In a part of Russian women with reproductive dysfunction belonging to group 2, the number of B-lymphocytes was approximately higher than 8.5%, which should be considered of high prognostic significance (AUROC = 0.968).

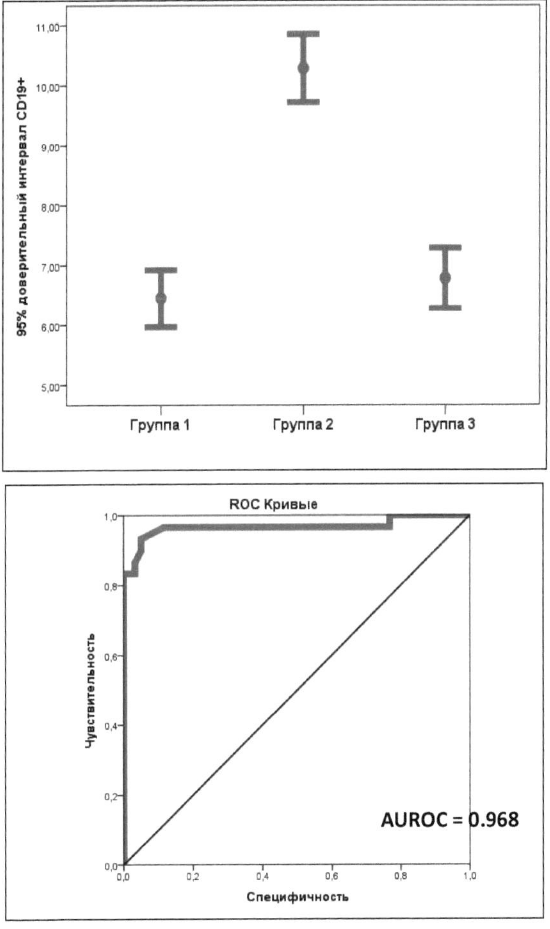

Figure 56. 95% confidence intervals of B-lymphocyte counts in the blood of Russian women of the study groups and ROC curve

the predictive value of the test
(green colour indicates the reference value area)

Thus, the studied immunophenotypic characteristics of lymphocytes almost in full (except for the number of CD3+ cells) can serve as markers of risk groups for the threat to women's reproductive health in the Russian population. It should be emphasised that all prognostically significant deviations of the above quantitative indicators do not exceed the physiological norm, but in case of their combination with each other they indicate the risk of reproductive disorders.

5.1.2 Levels of immunoglobulins of different classes and groups at risk of reproductive health problems of women in the Russian population

In this section of the study, the possible pathogenetic role of immunoglobulins of three classes (IgM, IgG, IgA) in the development of reproductive pathology in women of the Russian population was elucidated. The results of the study of imm noglobulin levels by individual groups are presented in Table 21 and Figure 57.

Table 21. Levels of immunoglobulins of different classes in blood women in the Russian population and study groups

Informative indicators	Median indicator [minimum, maximum]			p_1 p_2 p_3
	Group 1	Group 2	Group 3	
IgM (mg/ml)	1,2 [0,7; 1,9]	1,2 [0,2; 2,1]	1,2 [0,9; 1,8]	0,661 0,661 0,983
IgG (mg/ml)	9,8 [8,5; 12,1]	12,2 [10,7; 14,8]	9,9 [8,7; 12,0]	<0,001 <0,001 0,956

IgA (mg/ml)	2,0 [1,6; 2,5]	1,5 [0,9; 3,5]	2,1 [1,7; 2,5]	<0,001 <0,001 0,961

Note: p_1 - probability of data differences in groups 1 and 2; p_2 - probability of data differences in groups 2 and 3; p_3 - probability of data differences in groups 1 and 3; grey shows significance of differences ($p<0.05$) by Mann-Whitney test

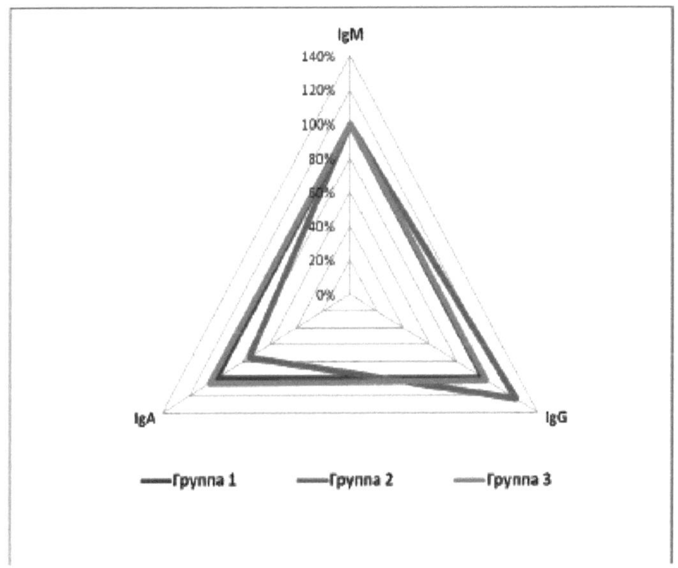

Figure 57. Percentages of deviation of immunoglobulin content of different classes in the blood of Russian women with reproductive disorders from that of healthy women

As can be seen from the table and figure, in the Russian population there are no intergroup differences in the level of IgM (the 95% confidence interval level was not analysed), therefore this immunoglobulin was not further analysed. For the other classes of immunoglobulins, there are significant deviations, but only in group 2.

Analysis of 95% confidence intervals of IgG level showed that it is quite informative in the group of 2 Russian women at a concentration of approximately above 11 mg/ml. As the results of ROC curves (Figure 58) showed, this indicator is highly prognostically significant for determining whether a woman belongs to a risk group for reproductive disorders, since the AUROC is 0.927.

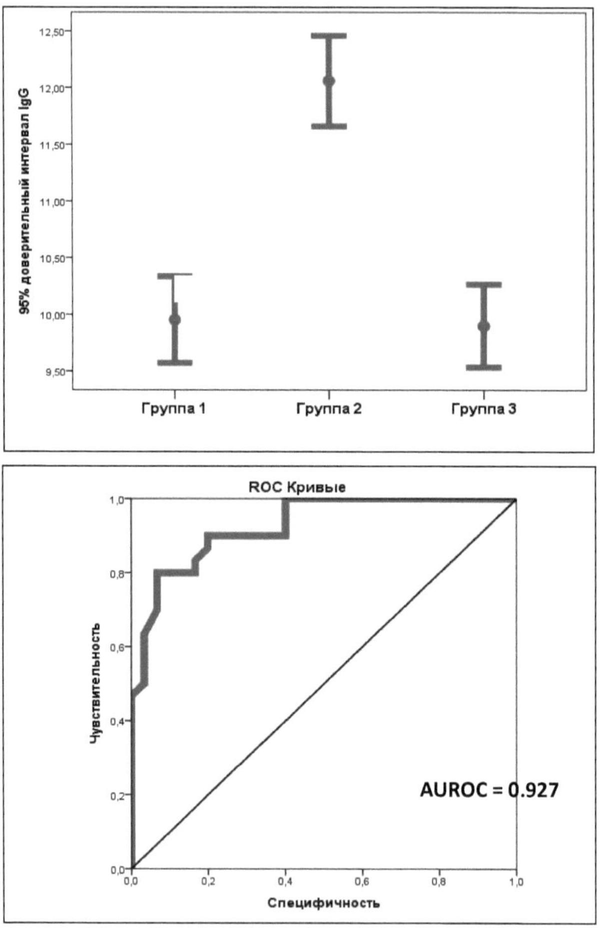

Figure 58. 95% confidence intervals of IgG levels in blood Russian women in the study groups and the ROC curve of the predictive value of the test
(green colour indicates the reference value area)

As for IgA levels, Figure 59 shows that this indicator decreased in the presence of reproductive dysfunction in the group of 2 Russian women, but the prognostic significance of this decrease was moderate in the population of Russian women, with an AUROC of only 0.711.

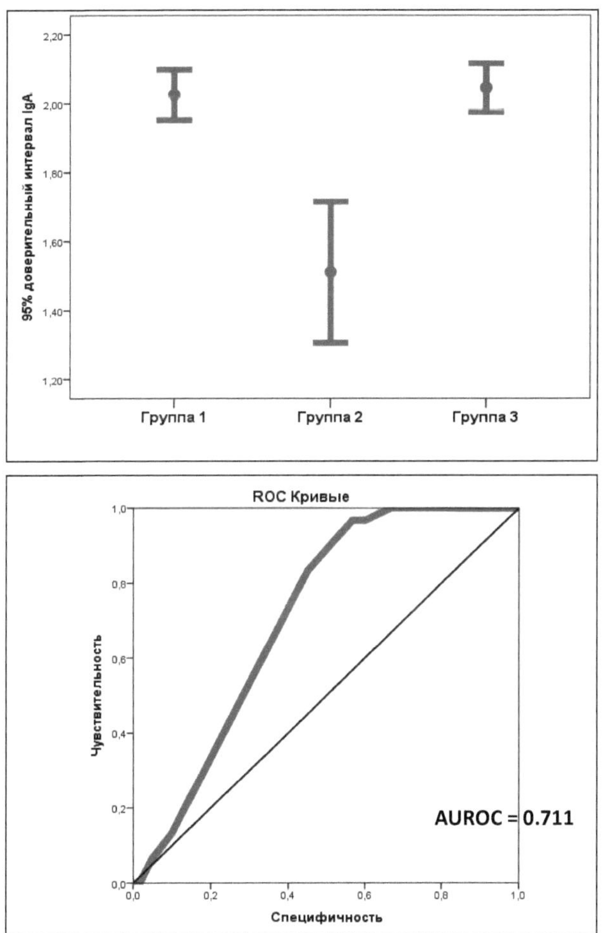

Figure 59. 95% confidence intervals of blood IgA levels Russian women in the study groups and the ROC curve of the predictive value of the test
(green colour indicates the reference value area)

Thus, among the three classes of immunoglobulins, only the level of IgG showed sufficient (high) prognostic significance, while IgM and IgA had no prognostic significance in terms of reproductive health disorders.

5.1.3 Antiphospholipid Reactions and Risk Groups for Reproductive Health Disorders among Women in the Russian Population

Antiphospholipid reactions as an autoimmune hypercoagulable state caused by antiphospholipid antibodies are closely associated with pregnancy pathology in a certain proportion of women with reproductive disorders. The objective of this section of the study was to analyse the traits of those groups of women in whom antiphospholipid reactions were associated with reproductive impairment in a population cluster approach to the problem. The results of such analyses are presented in Table 22 and Figure 60.

Table 22. Indices of antiphospholipid reaction in blood Russian women of different study groups

Informative indicators	Median indicator [minimum, maximum]			p_1 p_2 p_3
	Group 1	Group 2	Group 3	
IgG-antibodies to human phospholipids (units/ml)	3,1 [1,1; 4,5]	5,1 [3,6; 7,1]	3,1 [1,0; 4,2]	<0,001 <0,001 0,896
IgG-antibodies to β2-glycoprotein 1 (units/ml)	3,6 [1,2; 4,3]	6,6 [4,9; 8,5]	3,5 [1,6; 4,3]	<0,001 <0,001 0,560
IgG-antibodies to annexin V (units/ml)	1,9 [1,0; 4,2]	2,4 [1,5; 2,8]	2,0 [1,2; 4,0]	0,004 0,002 0,670
IgG-antibodies to prothrombin (units/ml)	3,8 [1,2; 8,6]	5,3 [3,9; 7,3]	3,0 [1,2; 8,0]	0,004 0,001 0,663

Lupus anticoagulant (units/ml)	0,8 [0,6; 1,1]	1,1 [0,6; 1,5]	0,9 [0,7; 1,1]	<0,001 <0,001 0,400
Lebetox test (min.)	1,3 [0,5; 3,7]	1,5 [1,0; 2,0]	1,4 [0,4; 3,7]	0,229 0,490 0,683

Note: p_1 - probability of data differences in groups 1 and 2; p_2 - probability of data differences in groups 2 and 3; p_3 - probability of data differences in groups 1 and 3; grey shows significance of differences ($p<0.05$) by Mann-Whitney test

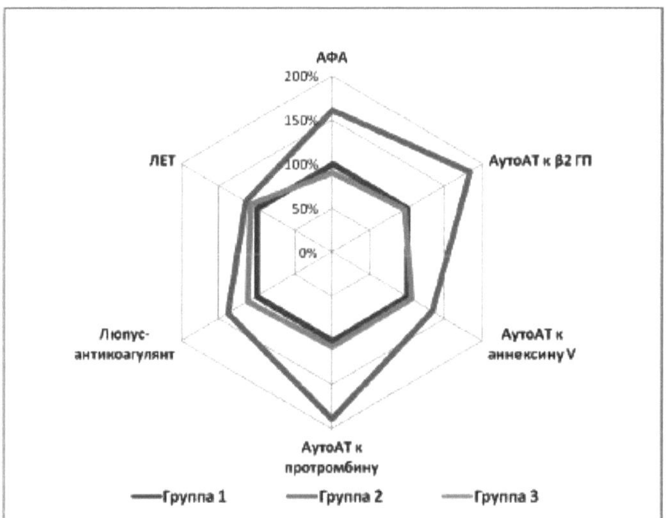

Figure 60. Percentages of deviation of antiphospholipid indices reactions in the blood of Russian women with reproductive disorders from those of healthy women

(* - differences between the values of indicators are statistically reliable)

As follows from the table and figure, laboratory signs of antiphospho lipid reactions allow us to identify their presence in a certain cohort of women belonging to the Russian population.

In Russian women, an increase in the values of antiphospholipid reaction indicators was noted in group 2 with reproductive health disorders. In this group the levels of total autoantibodies of IgG class to human phospholipids, IgG-autoantibodies to β_2 -glycoprotein, annexin V, prothrombin, blood content of lupus anticoagulant increased significantly. All this allows us to consider that these features characterise group 2 in the Russian population as a risk group.

To clarify the possibility of using the established deviations from control as markers of reproductive health disorders in the named groups, their 95% confidence intervals were determined and ROC curves were constructed (Figures 61-65).

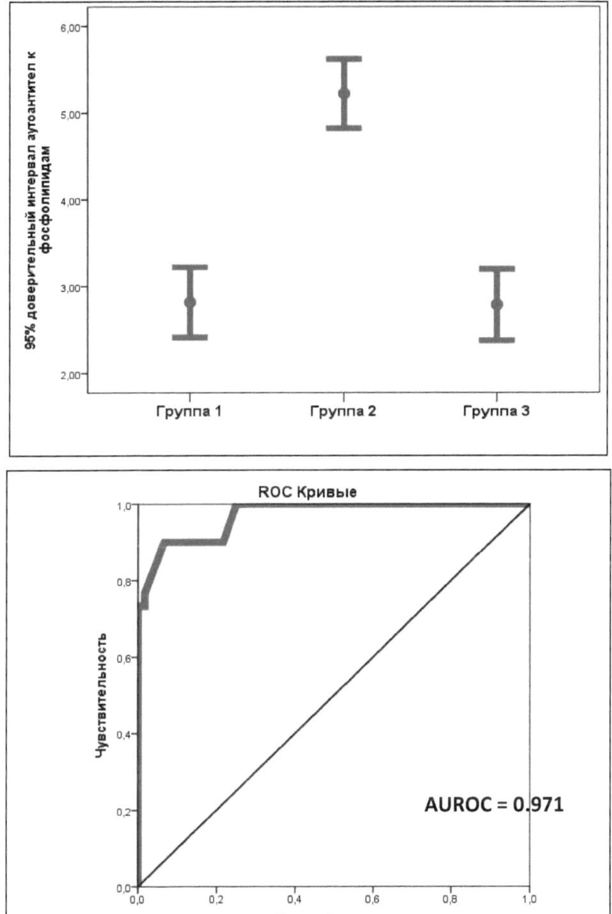

Figure 61. 95% confidence intervals of autoantibodies to phospholipids in the blood of Russian women of the study groups and ROC curve the predictive value of the test

(green colour indicates the reference value area)

Figure 61 shows 95% confidence intervals and prognostic significance for the level of total autoantibodies to a set of phospholipids. An increase in the values of this indicator approximately above 4 U/ml was noted for group 2 of Russian women, with an AUROC value of 0.971, indicating the high prognostic value of this test in detecting disorders of female reproductive health.

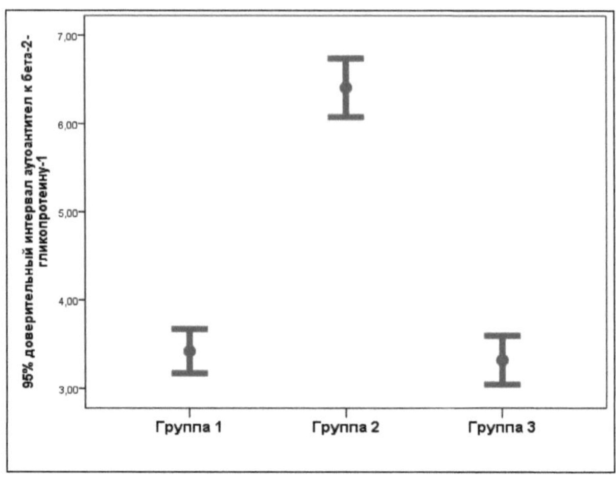

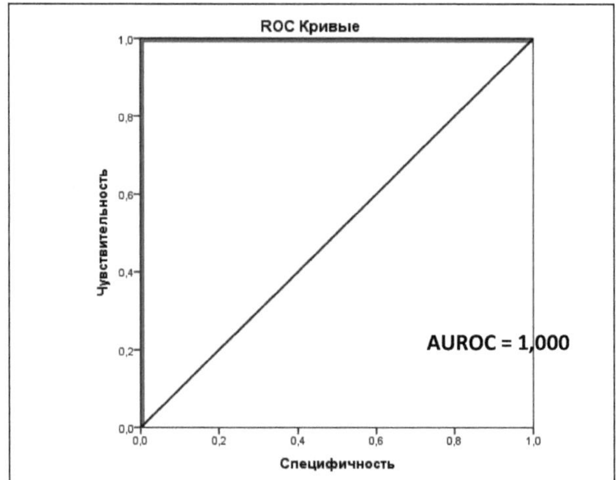

Figure 62. 95% confidence intervals of autoantibodies to β_2 -glycoprotein-1 in the blood of Russian women of the studied groups and ROC curve of the predictive value of the test

(green colour indicates the reference value area)

The increased level of IgG autoantibodies to β_2 -glycoprotein in the group of 2 Russian women showed a particularly high prognostic significance, close to absolute (AUROC = 1.0). The value of this indicator in the risk group above 4.5 U/ml was indicative of impaired reproductive function, as clearly shown in Figure 62.

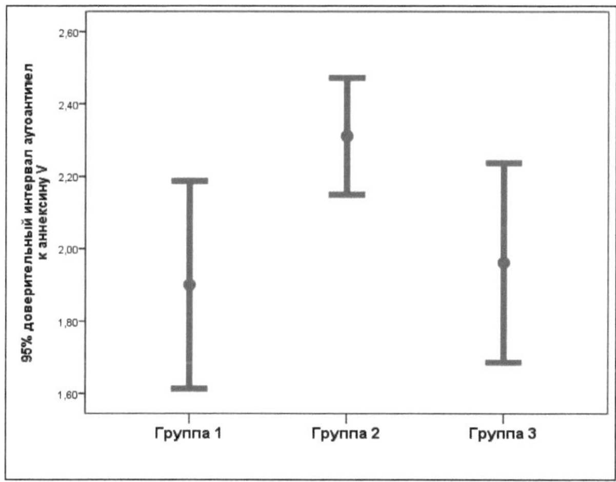

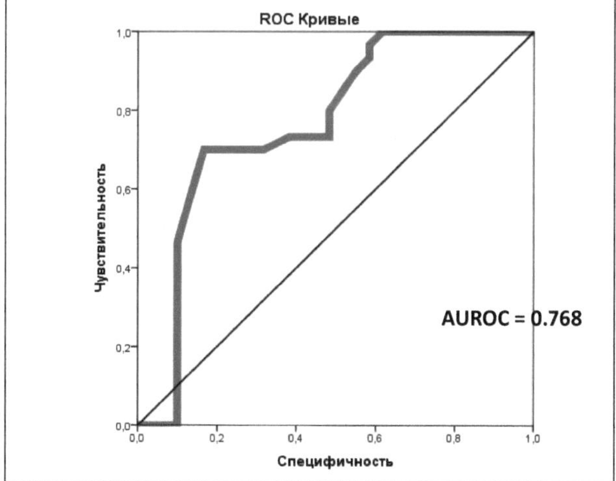

Figure 63. 95% confidence intervals of autoantibodies to annexin V in the blood of Russian women of the study groups and ROC curve

the predictive value of the test
(green colour indicates the reference value area)

At the same time, the increase in the level of IgG-autoantibodies to annexin V (Figure 63), although it showed, according to Table 12, a reliable deviation from the indicators of healthy women in group 2 of the Russian population, from the point of view of prognostic significance was moderate (AUROC = 0.768) and cannot claim to be a marker of reproductive disorders.

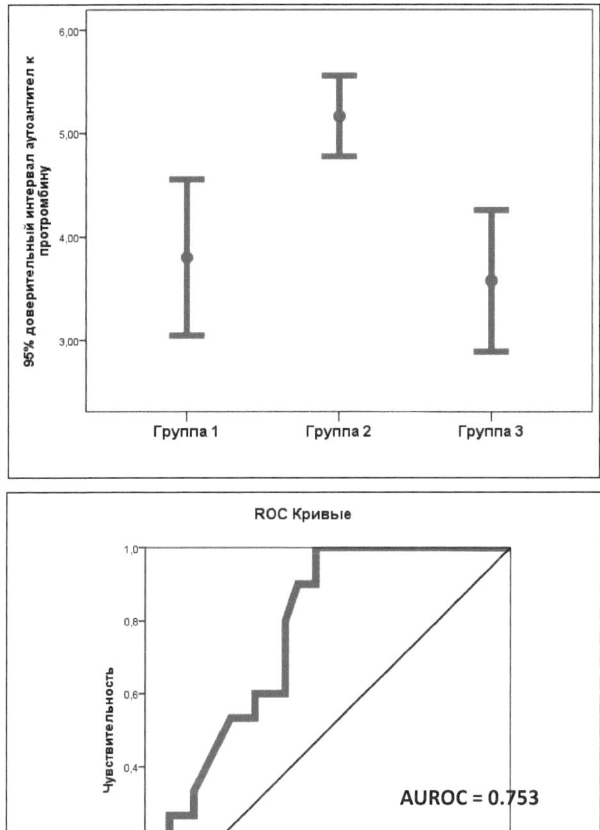

Figure 64. 95% confidence intervals of autoantibodies to prothrombin in the blood of Russian women of the studied groups and the ROC curve of the predictive value of the test

(green colour indicates the reference value area)

Figure 64 shows the level of IgG-autoantibodies to prothrombin in the studied groups. In group 2 of the population of Russian women, the increase in this indicator was registered with moderate prognostic significance (AUROC = 0.753), which made it inappropriate to use it to determine whether a woman belongs to a risk group for reproductive failure.

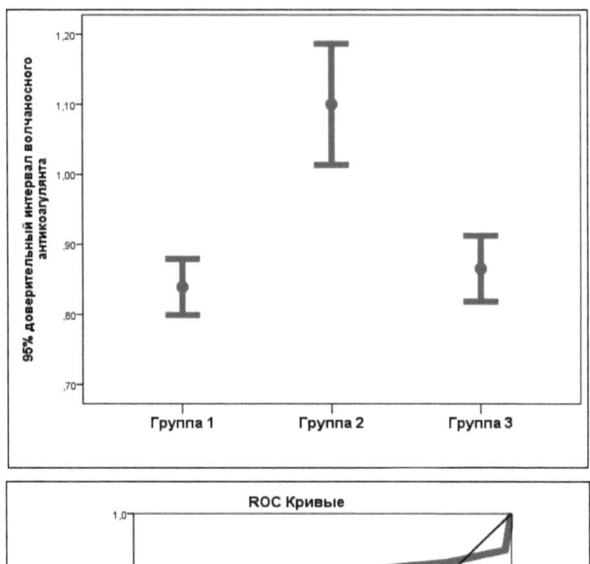

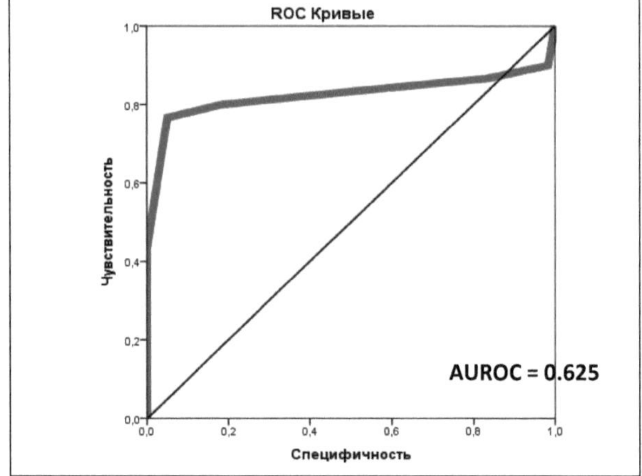

Figure 65. 95% confidence intervals of lupus anticoagulant in the blood of Russian women of the studied groups and the ROC curve of the predictive value of the test

(green colour indicates the reference value area)

The lupus test for lupus anticoagulant (Figure 65) in the groups with reproductive health problems had moderate prognostic significance with AUROC = 0.625, making it difficult to use as a marker of risk groups. As for the lebetox test for lupus anticoagulant, this indicator did not yield intergroup significant differences and for this reason was not analysed for prognostic significance.

Thus, antiphospholipid reactions, indeed, accompany a certain risk group (2) in the population of Russian women, and its laboratory signs may serve as markers of reproductive disorders. Among the markers, the leading significance in Russian women belongs to the increase in the level of IgG-autoantibodies to phospholipids and β_2 - glycoprotein-1.

5.1.4 Ranges of prognostically important values of indicators immune status in a risk group of Russian women

The aim of this research section was to clarify the ranges of prognostically important values of immunological markers of risk group 2 in the population of Russian women. For this purpose, we compared the borderline values of 95% confidence intervals of all the markers obtained by study group, taking into account their standard deviations. The results of this study are presented in Table 23.

When the prognostic values in group 3 exceeded the 95% confidence intervals in the other groups or, conversely, exceeded them, the lower or upper limits of these intervals for the prognostically significant indicators and the upper/lower limits for the same indicators in the other two groups were compared, respectively, with the maximum or minimum value among those in the comparison groups taken as the boundary of the prognostically significant range.

Table 23. Borderline values and prognostically significant values for immunological parameters in women of the Russian population in the study groups

Informative indicators	Upper/ lower boundary for groups 1	Upper/ lower boundary for groups 2	Upper/ lower boundary for groups of 3	Prognostically significant range values in group 3
T-helpers (CD3+CD4+), %	max 35,7	min 35,7	max 34,8	> 35,7%
Cytotoxic T-lymphocytes (CD3+CD8+),%	max 19,7	min 21,7	max 20,2	> 20,2%
ECT (CD3+CD56+), %	max 4,2	min 3,6	max 4,2	> 4,2%
Natural killer cells (CD16+CD56+),	max 14,6	min 14,8	max 13,8	> 14,6%
B-lymphocytes (CD19+), %	max 9,3	min 8,5	max 9,3	> 9,3%
IgG, mg/ml	max 10,6	min 10,6	max 10,2	> 10.6 mg/ml
IgG-antibodies to phospholipids, units/ml	max 3,6	min 3,6	max 3,3	> 3.6 units/ml
IgG-antibodies to β_2 - glycoprotein-1,	max 4,8	min 4,8	max 4,5	> 4.8 units/ml

Note: grey indicates borderline prognostically significant value

As follows from the table, prognostically significant values have been established, allowing us to determine the borderline values of the indicators, beyond which they can be considered markers of reproductive disorders. In cases where the values of the indicator were within the prognostically significant range, especially in the absence of obstetric history, the woman could be assigned to the appropriate risk group.

5.2 Immune status and risk groups for disorders

5.2.1 Phenotypic characterisation of lymphocytes and groups at risk of reproductive health problems women in the Tajik population

The results of the study of immune status abnormalities associated with reproductive health disorders in the population of Tajik women of different group affiliation are presented in Table 24 and Figure 66.

Table 24.

Percentage of lymphocytes of different phenotypes in the blood of Tajik women of different study groups

Informative indicators	Median indicator [minimum, maximum]			p_1 p_2 p_3
	Group 5	Group 6	Group 7	
T-lymphocytes are. CD3+	67,4 [64,6; 75,2]	59,3 [55,6; 62,4]	66,4 [62,8; 71,1]	<0,001 <0,001 0,854
T-helper cells CD3+CD4+	33,0 [29,9; 39,8]	36,5 [33,7; 39,2]	33,2 [30,7; 35,3]	<0,001 <0,001 0,712
Cytotoxic T-lymphocytes - CD3+CD8+	21,2 [13,2; 23,3]	19,2 [17,1; 21,5]	21,8 [19,1; 24,3]	<0,001 <0,001 0,587
EKT - CD3+CD56+	3,2 [2,6; 7,6]	9,5 [7,6; 12,1]	3,2 [1,7; 4,4]	<0,001 <0,001 0,966
Natural killers - CD16+CD56+	10,4 [3,2; 11,6]	19,5 [17,2; 22,9]	10,4 [8,5; 12,4]	<0,001 <0,001 0,938
B-lymphocytes - CD19+	12,6 [11,1; 15,5]	15,8 [14,2; 19,9]	12,8 [9,9; 16,7]	<0,001 <0,001 0,628

Note: p_1 - probability of data differences in groups 5 and 6; p_2 - probability of data differences in groups 6 and 7; p_3 - probability of data differences in groups 5 and 7; grey shows significance of differences ($p<0.05$) by Mann-Whitney test

As the data obtained show, the nature of changes in immunophenotypic indicators using the population cluster approach in Tajik women are fundamentally different from those in the Russian population.

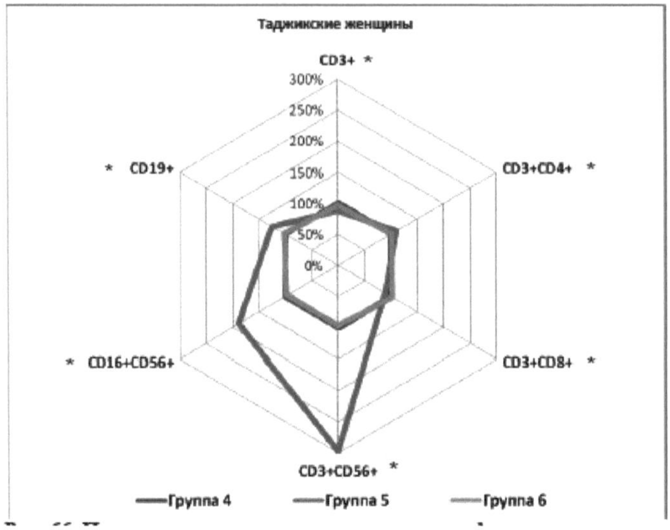

Figure 66. Percentages of deviation of the content of lymphocytes of different phenotypes in the blood of women with reproductive disorders from those of healthy women
(* - differences between the values of indicators are statistically reliable)

In particular, in the population of Tajik women, the main immunophenotypic shifts were observed in the same group in which hormonal shifts were registered - in group 6. The main emphasis in the degree of deviation from the indicators of healthy women fell, first of all, on the lymphocytes of the innate immune response, which take part in the realisation of reproductive function - EC (CD16+CD56+) and ECP (CD3+CD56+). In parallel, the number of B-lymphocytes increased, which coincided with the previously reported increase in the levels of autoantibodies to thyroid proteins in this category of women.

The data obtained created a prerequisite for the creation of a system of immunophenotypic markers of reproductive health disorders in women in group 6 of the Tajik population by analysing all tested indicators on the basis of their 95% confidence intervals and their corresponding ROC curves (Figures 67-72).

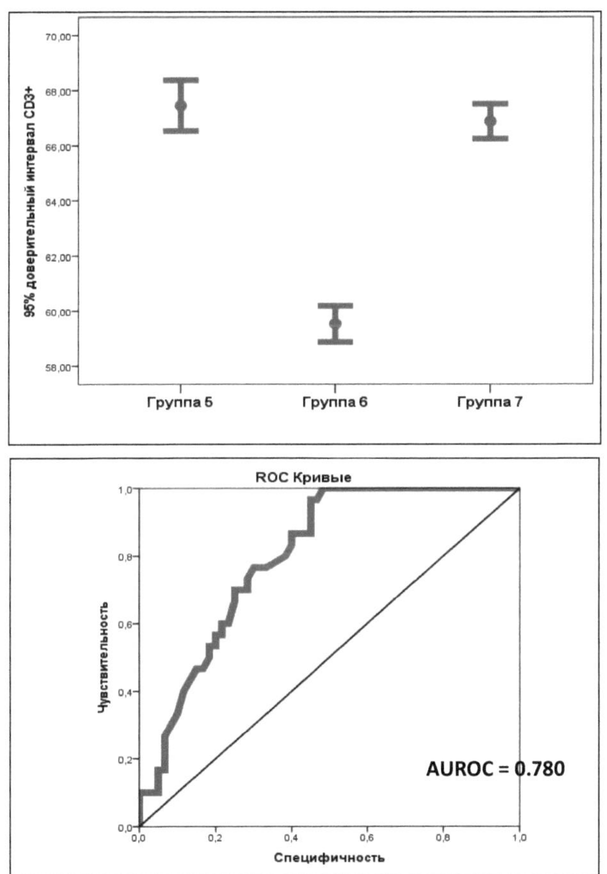

Figure 67. 95% confidence intervals of T-lymphocyte counts in the blood of Tajik women of the study groups and ROC curve the predictive value of the test
(green colour indicates the reference value area)

Figure 67 shows the results of determining the 95% confidence intervals of the relative number of T-lymphocytes in the blood by individual groups in the population of Tajik women. Thus, the relative number of T-lymphocytes with CD3+ phenotype was reduced in group 6, but this indicator had moderate prognostic significance.

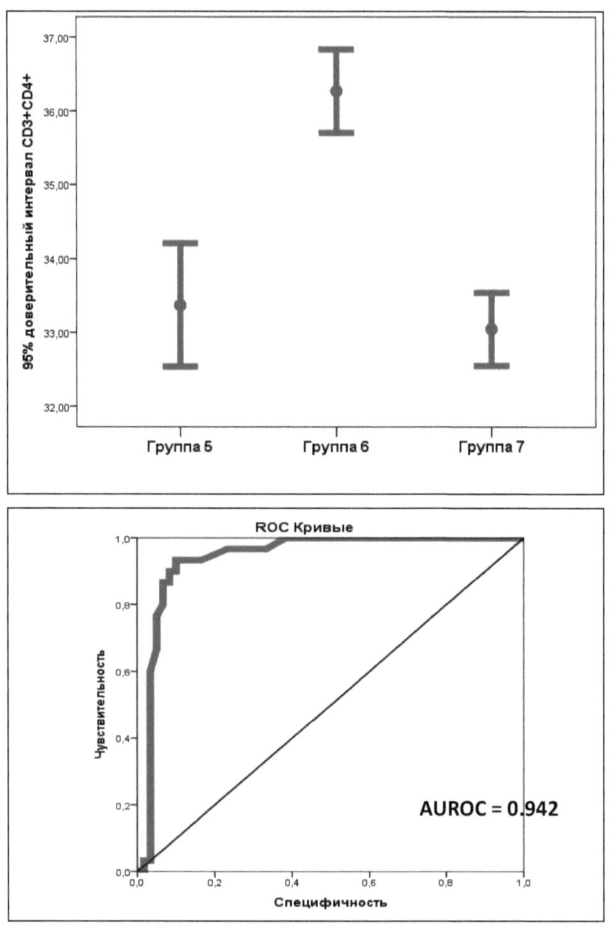

Figure 68. 95% confidence intervals of the number of T-helper cells
in the blood of women in the study groups and ROC curves the predictive value of the test
(green colour indicates the reference value area)

Figure 68 shows the 95% confidence limits for one of the main subpopulations of T-lymphocytes - T-helper cells (CD3+CD4+). The relative number of these cells was >35% in the group of 6 Tajik women with impaired reproductive function, and the prognostic significance of the test was high, as the AUROC value was at 0.942.

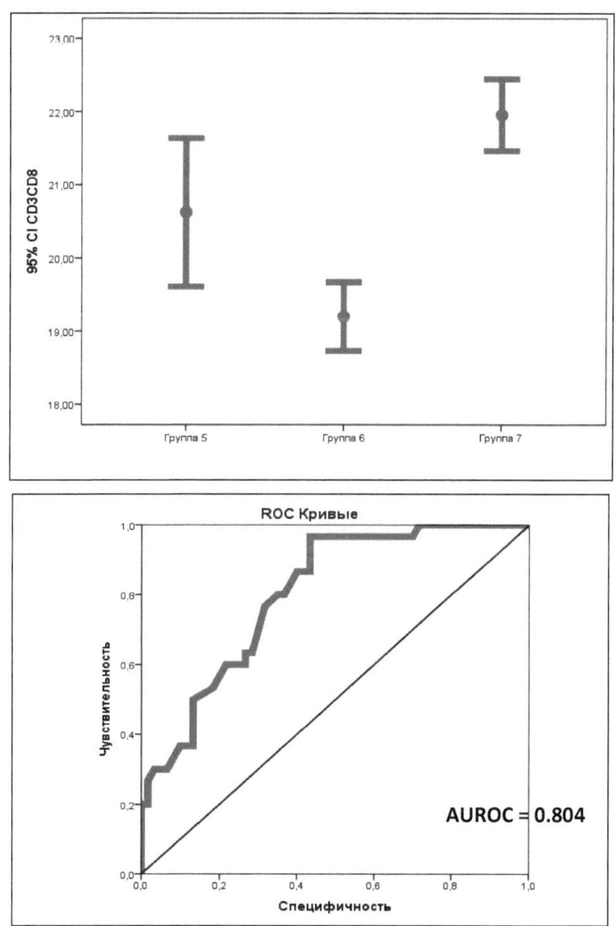

Figure 69. 95% confidence intervals of the number of cytotoxic T-lymphocytes in the blood of women of the studied groups and ROC curves of the predictive value of the test
(green colour indicates the reference value area)

The relative number of cytotoxic T lymphocytes (CD3+CD8+) was highly prognostically significant (AUROC = 0.804), as shown in Figure 69. In group 6 of the Tajik population with reproductive health problems, the number of CTLs had such significance with values < 19.5 per cent.

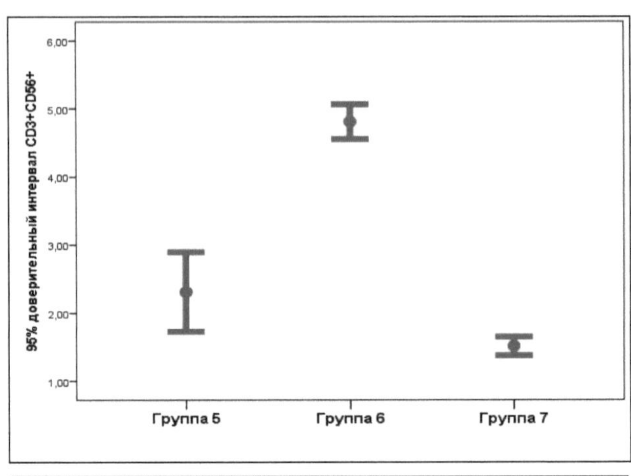

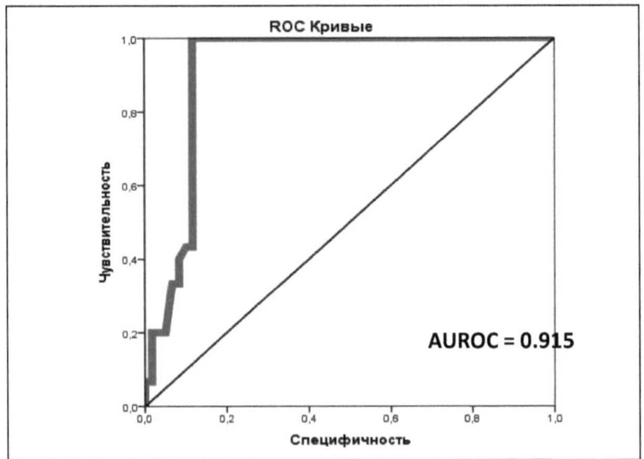

Figure 70. 95% confidence intervals of the number of ECTs in blood
Tajik women in the study groups and ROC curve the predictive value of the test
(green colour indicates the reference value area)

High prognostic significance (AUROC = 0.915) was demonstrated by the percentage of ECT among blood lymphocytes (Figure 70). In the Tajik population of women in group 6, this indicator had the characteristics of a marker of the reproductive disorders risk group when its value increased above 4%.

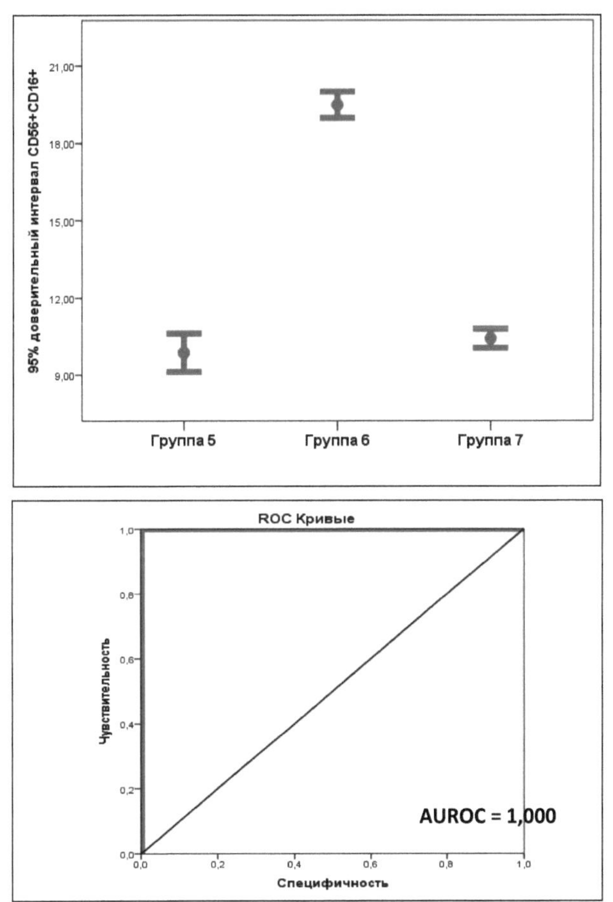

Figure 71. 95% confidence intervals of the number of natural killer cells in the blood of Tajik women of the study groups and ROC curve the predictive value of the test

(green colour indicates the reference value area)

The relative number of natural killer cells when performing phenotypic analyses of blood lymphocytes proved to be the most important prognostic feature, as the AUROC value, which is a quantitative criterion for such significance, was close to absolute and was 1.0. The percentage of EC among blood lymphocytes was >15% in group 6 of the Tajik population (Figure 71).

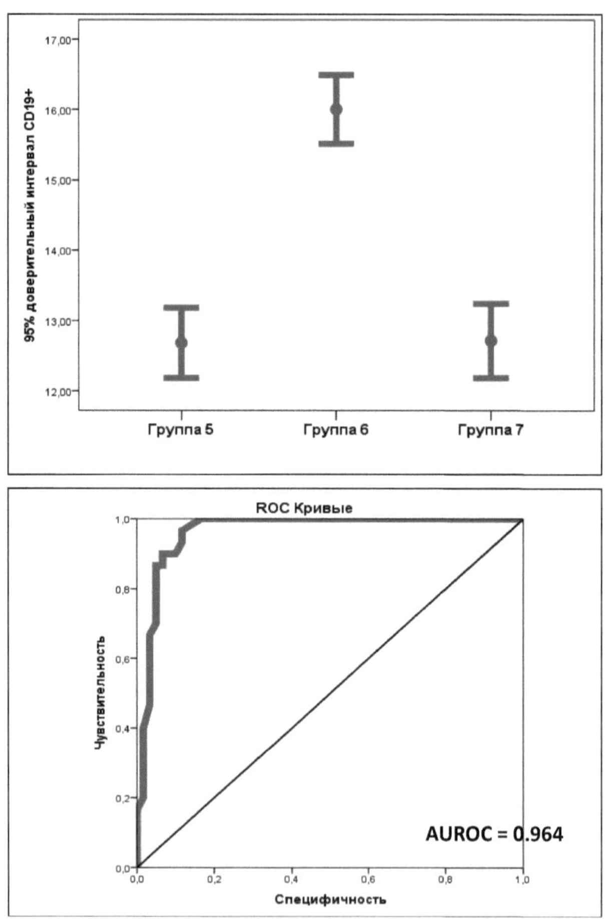

Figure 72. 95% confidence intervals of B-lymphocyte counts

in the blood of Tajik women of the study groups and ROC curve the predictive value of the test

(green colour indicates the reference value area)

The B-lymphocyte content in the blood of women with reproductive disorders can also claim to be a marker of such disorders (Figure 72). In a part of Tajik women with reproductive disorders in Group 6, a B-lymphocyte count higher than 14.5% should be considered of high prognostic significance (AUROC = 0.964).

Thus, the studied immunophenotypic characteristics of lymphocytes almost in full (except for the number of CD3+ cells) can serve as markers of risk groups for the threat to women's reproductive health in the Tajik population. It should be stressed that all prognostically significant deviations of the above quantitative indicators do not exceed the physiological norm, but in case of their combination with each other indicate the risk of reproductive disorders at the preclinical stage.

5.2.2 Levels of immunoglobulins of different classes and groups at risk of reproductive health problems women in the Tajik population

In this section of the research, the possible role of serum immunoglobulins of three classes (IgM, IgG, IgA) in the development of reproductive disorders at the preclinical stage in women of the Tajik population was elucidated.

The results of such a study to identify deviations of immunoglobulin levels within reference values in Tajik women with preserved and impaired reproductive function are presented in Table 25 and Figure 73.

In Tajik women, reliable deviations from the indicators of healthy women appear in group 6 for all classes of immunoglobulins.

Table 25. Levels of immunoglobulins of different classes in blood
women in the Tajik population of different study groups

Informative indicators	Median indicator [minimum,			p_1 p_2
	Groups of	Groups of	Groups of	
IgM (mg/ml)	1,0 [0,1; 2,5]	1,6 [1,0; 1,9]	1,1 [0,4; 2,7]	0,001 <0,001
IgG (mg/ml)	12,5 [11,0;	14,4 [12,9;	12,2 [10,2;	<0,001 <0,001
IgA (mg/ml)	1,4 [0,5; 3,0]	0,8 [0,3; 2,0]	1,3 [0,1; 3,0]	<0,001 0,001

Note: p_1 - probability of data differences in groups 5 and 6; p_2 - probability of data differences in groups 6 and 7; p_3 - probability of data differences in groups 5 and 7; grey shows significance of differences ($p<0.05$) by Mann-Whitney test

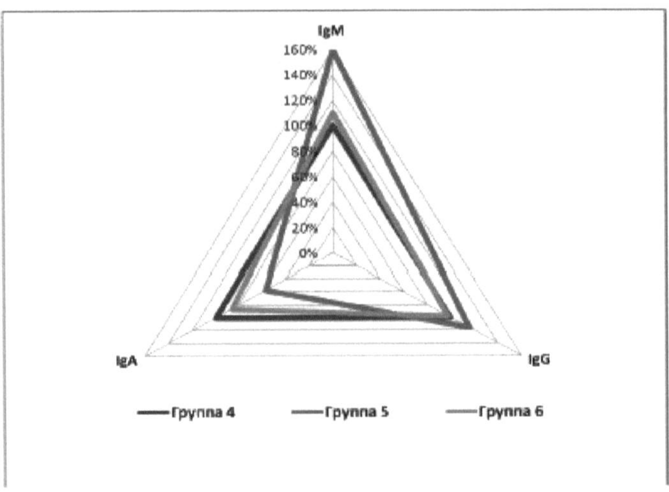

Figure 73. Percentages of deviation of immunoglobulin content

of different classes in the blood of Tajik women with reproductive disorders from that of healthy women

Next, the 95% confidence intervals of the levels of all immunoglobulins in the groups were compared and the prognostic significance of each of them in group 6, assessed as a risk group for reproductive failure in Tajik women, was determined by plotting ROC curves and calculating AUROC (Figures 74-76).

Analysis of 95% confidence intervals and ROC curves for IgM level (Figure 74) shows that in the population of Tajik women this indicator increases in group 6 and shows moderate prognostic significance (AUROC = 0.784). We recognise this level of predictive value as insufficient for the indicator to be used as a marker of reproductive health impairment.

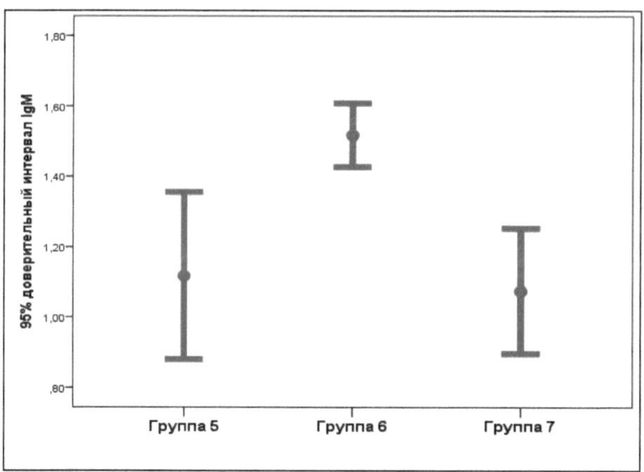

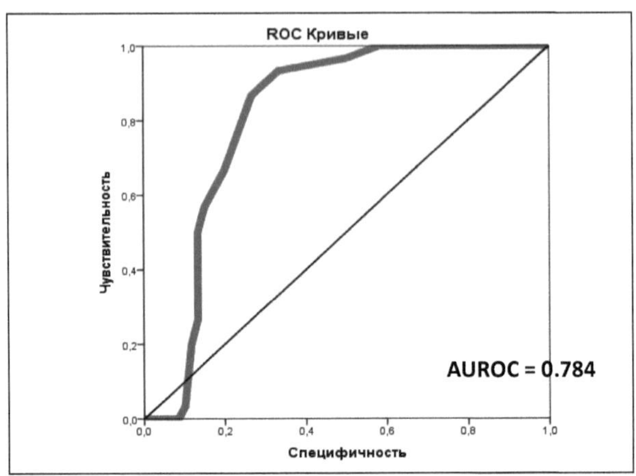

Figure 74. 95% confidence intervals of blood IgM levels Tajik women in the study groups and the ROC curve of the predictive value of the test
(green colour indicates the reference value area)

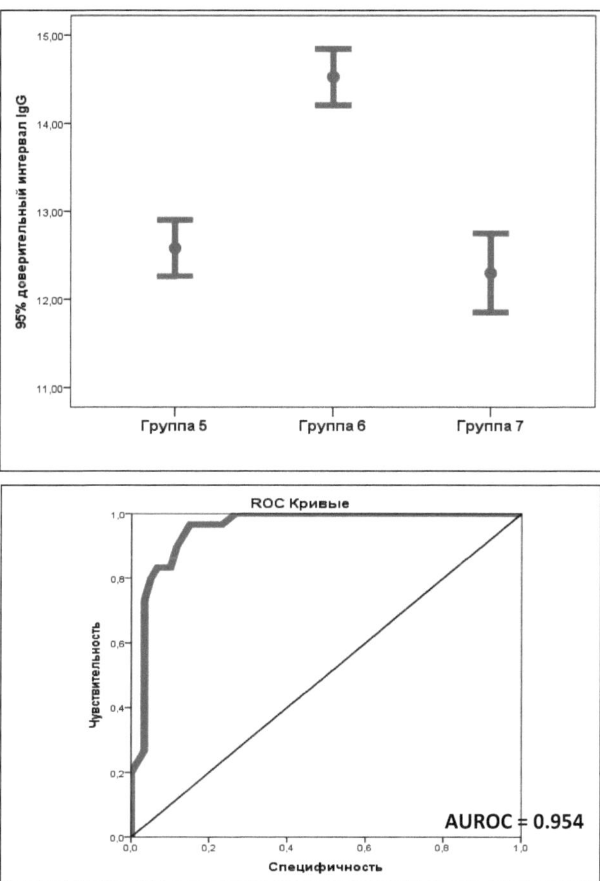

Figure 75. 95% confidence intervals of IgG levels in blood Tajik women in the study groups and the ROC curve of the predictive value of the test
(green colour indicates the reference value area)

From this point of view, the level of IgG as a potential marker of reproductive disorders is favourable (Figure 75). An increase in the 95% confidence interval of this immunoglobulin in the group of 6 Tajik women above 14 mg/ml is highly prognostically significant, as AUROC is characterised by a value of 0.954.

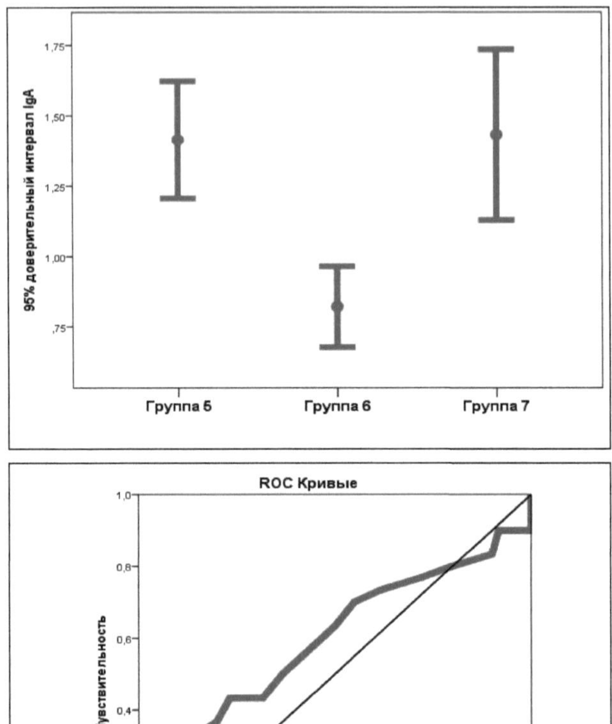

Figure 76. 95% confidence intervals of blood IgA levels Tajik women in the study groups and the ROC curve of the predictive value of the test

(green colour indicates the reference value area)

As for the IgA level, Figure 76 shows that this indicator decreased in the presence of reproductive disorders in the group of 6 Tajik women, but the prognostic significance of this decrease was practically absent in the population of Tajik women (AUROC = 0.592).

Thus, as in the population of Russian women, among the three classes of immunoglobulins, only the level of IgG had sufficient (high) prognostic significance as a marker of reproductive disorders in Tajik women.

5.2.3 Antiphospholipid reactions and risk groups Reproductive health disorders among women in Tajik populations

The objective of this section of the study was to analyse the traits of those groups of women in the Tajik population in whom antiphospholipid reactions were associated with reproductive disorders using a population-cluster approach to the problem.

The results of the analysis of autoimmune features of antiphospholipid reactions in the Tajik population of women are presented in Table 27 and Figure 77.

Table 27. Indices of antiphospholipid syndrome in blood Tajik women of different study groups

Informative indicators	**Median indicator [minimum, maximum]**			p_1 p_2 p_3
	Group 5	**Group 6**	**Group 7**	
1	2	3	4	5
IgG-antibodies to human phospholipids (units/ml)	6,6 [5,0; 9,0]	6,5 [5,0; 8,1]	11,6 [9,0; 13,8]	0,974 <0,001 <0,001
IgG-antibodies to β2-glycoprotein 1 (units/ml)	7,2 [6,1; 8,6]	7,2 [6,0; 8,6]	11,0 [10,1; 12,6]	0,831 <0,001 <0,001
1	**2**	**3**	**4**	**5**
IgG-antibodies to annexin V (units/ml)	4,5 [1,9; 7,5]	4,6 [2,4; 6,2]	4,6 [3,5; 6,3]	0,749 0,149 0,094
IgG-antibodies to prothrombin (units/ml)	6,8 [4,7; 8,7]	6,6 [4,7; 8,7]	11,0 [9,0; 13,6]	0,700 <0,001 <0,001
Lupus anticoagulant (units/ml)	1,1 [0,1; 1,6]	1,1 [0,1; 1,6]	1,1 [0,1; 3,9]	0,613 0,786 0,526

Lebetox test (min.)	1,8 [0,8; 2,6]	1,8 [1,0; 2,5]	2,2 [0,1; 4,2]	0,811 0,006 0,009

Note: p_1 - probability of data differences in groups 5 and 6; p_2 - probability of data differences in groups 6 and 7; p_3 - probability of data differences in groups 5 and 7; grey shows significance of differences ($p<0.05$) by Mann-Whitney test

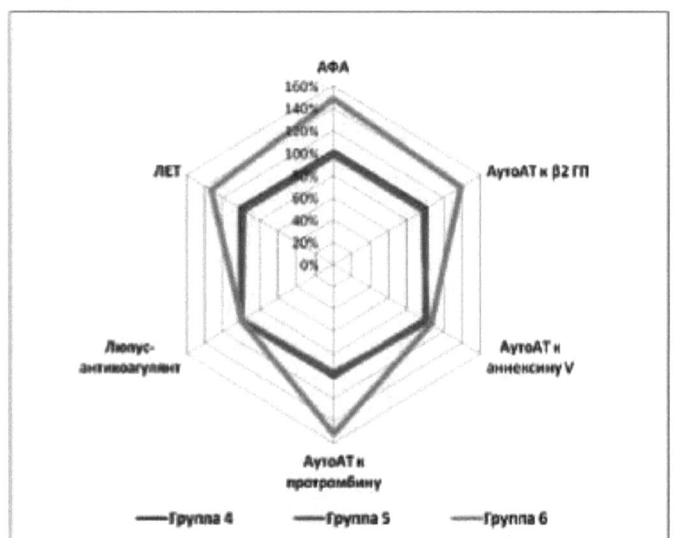

Figure 77. Percentages of deviation of antiphospholipid reaction indicators in the blood of Tajik women with reproductive disorders from those of healthy women

(* - differences between the values of indicators are statistically reliable)

As follows from the table and figure, deviations of laboratory indicators in the direction of signs of antiphospholipid reactions, although within the range of reference values, allow to identify their presence in a certain cohort of women belonging to the Tajik population.

The results showed that in Tajik women the list of deviations of antiphospholipid reactions signs from the indicators of healthy women extended to all autoimmune parameters, except for IgG autoantibodies to annexin V and lupus anticoagulant determined in the lupus test. In other words, the levels of IgG class autoantibodies to human phospholipids, β_2 -glycoprotein-1, prothrombin, as well as blood clotting time in the lebetox test remained promising for further investigation as markers of reproductive health disorders. All the described abnormalities were noted only in group 7 with reproductive disorders, in which no abnormalities in hormonal or immunophenotypic shifts were recorded by previous studies. To clarify the possibility of using the established significant deviations from the control as markers of reproductive health disorders in the above groups, as well as for other indicators, the 95% confidence intervals of all the indicators recognised as informative were determined and ROC-curves were constructed with AUROC calculation, as shown in Figures 78-81.

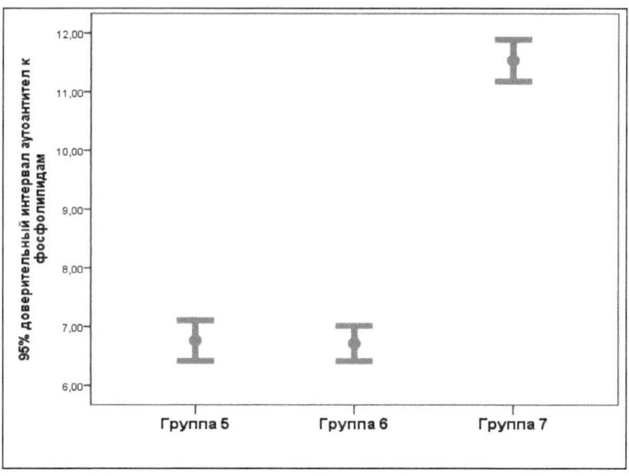

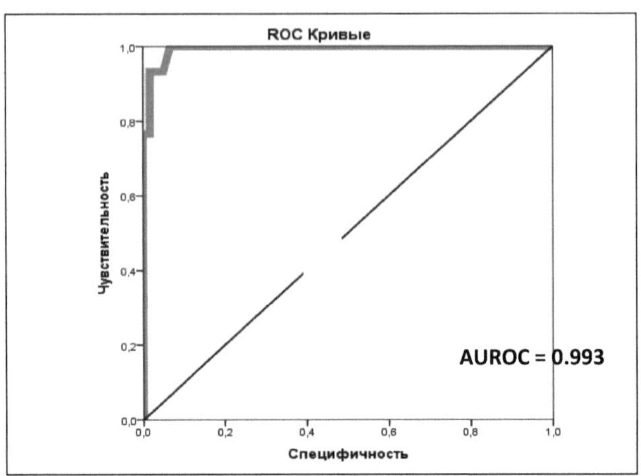

Figure 78. 95% confidence intervals of IgG autoantibodies to phospholipids in the blood of Tajik women of the study groups and the ROC curve of the predictive value of the test
(pink colour indicates the reference value area)

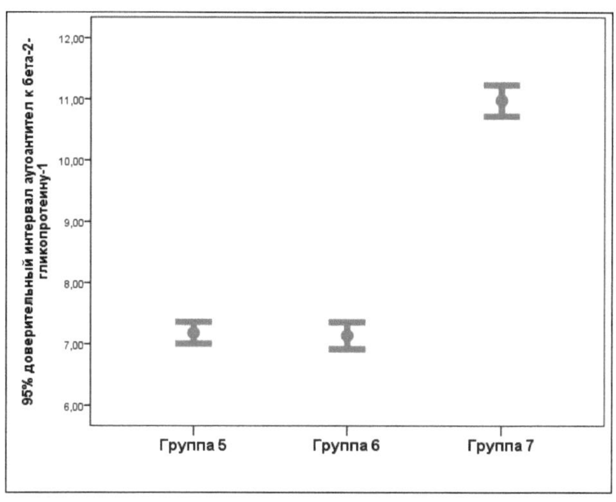

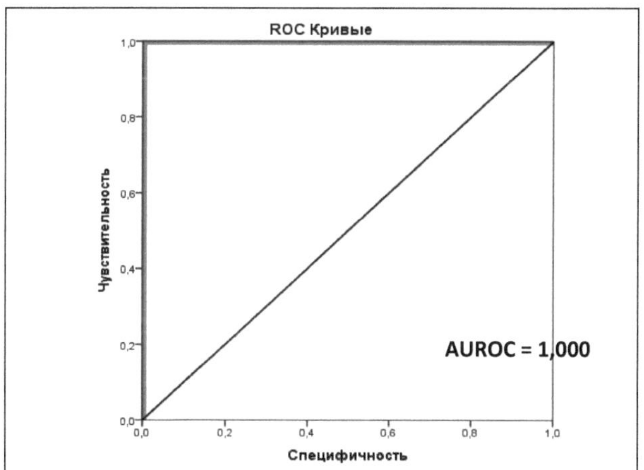

Figure 79. 95% confidence intervals of IgG autoantibodies to β_2 -glycoprotein in the blood of Tajik women of the studied groups and ROC curve of the predictive value of the test
(pink colour indicates the reference value area)

Thus, Figure 78 shows 95% confidence intervals and prognostic significance for the level of total IgG autoantibodies to a set of phospholipids. In the group of 7 Tajik women, this indicator deviated significantly from the values obtained in the other two study groups. Its values over the range of 95% confidence interval were approximately higher than 9 U/ml, and the degree of prognostic significance of the increased range of total autoantibodies to phospholipids should be recognised in Tajik women as very high with AUROC value equal to 0.993.

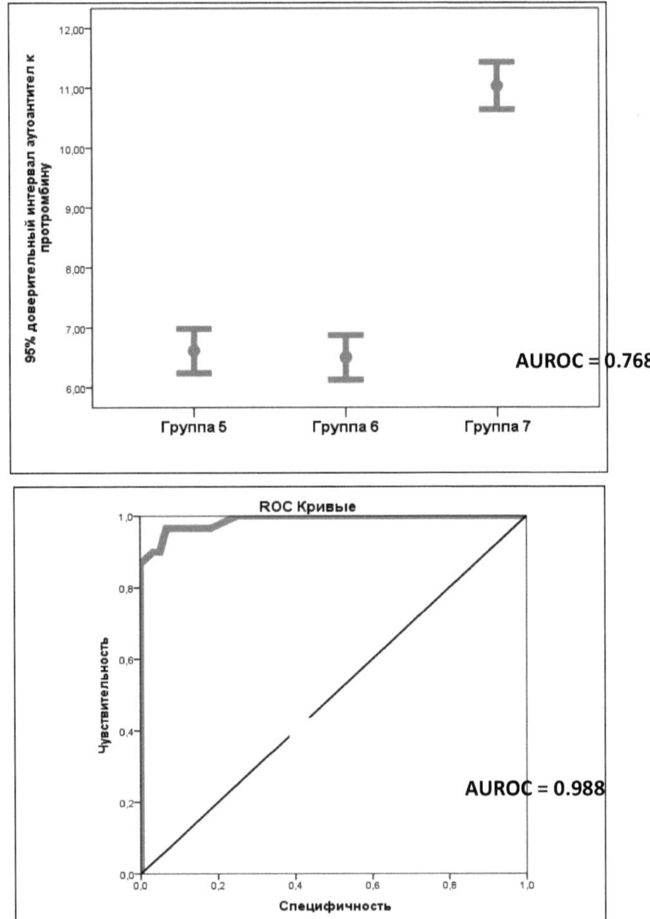

Figure 80. 95% confidence intervals of IgG autoantibodies to prothrombin in the blood of Tajik women of the study groups and ROC curve of the predictive value of the test
(pink colour indicates the reference value area)

Very high prognostic significance, close to absolute (AUROC = 1.0), was demonstrated in group 7 of Tajik population by the increased level of autoantibodies to β_2 -glycoprotein, the value of this indicator, indicating impaired reproductive function, in the named group was > 9 U/ml, as shown in Figure 79.

Figure 80 shows the 95% confidence intervals of IgG prothrombin autoantibodies in the study groups in the Tajik population. In group 7, a value of > 8 U/ml with a very high predictive value (AUROC = 0.988) indicated possible reproductive health impairment.

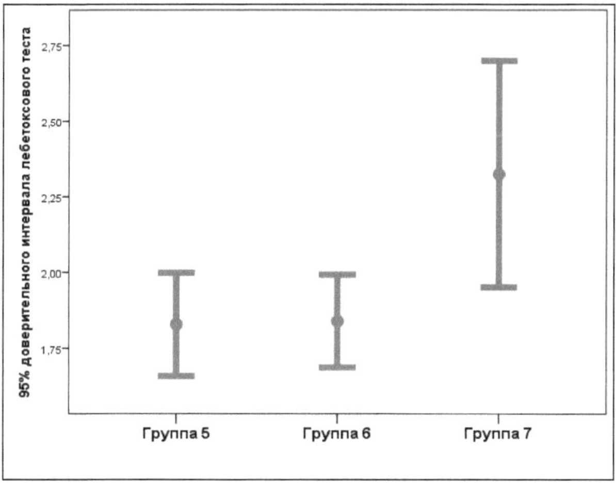

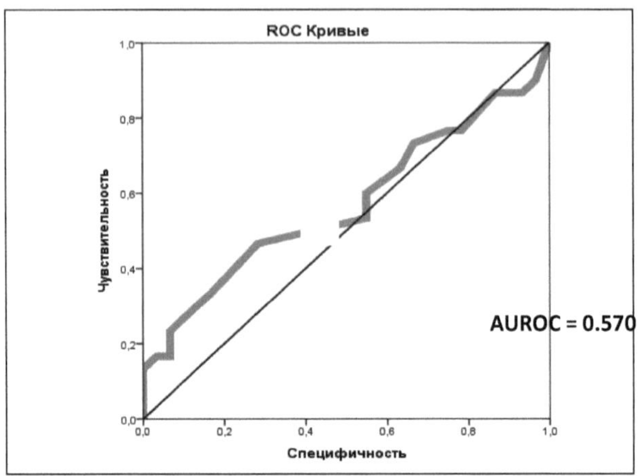

Figure 81. 95% confidence intervals of the lebetox test in the blood of Tajik women in the study groups and ROC curve of the predictive value of the test
(pink colour indicates the reference value area)

The lebetox test (Figure 81) in group 7 with reproductive health disorders did not have prognostic significance (AUROC = 0.570) in the population of Tajik women with possible reproductive health disorders and therefore we did not use it as a marker of the risk group for reproductive disorders.

Thus, antiphospholipid reactions, indeed, accompany certain risk groups (group 7) in the population of Tajik women, and their signs can serve as markers of reproductive disorders, according to our data, among them the leading importance belongs to the levels of IgG-autoantibodies to phospholipids, β_2 -glycoprotein-1, prothrombin.

5.2.4 Ranges of prognostically important values of indicators immune status in at-risk groups of Tajik women

The objective of this section of the study was to clarify the ranges of prognostically important values of immunological markers of two risk groups - 6 and 7 - in the population of Tajik women. For this purpose, the borderline values of 95% confidence intervals of all obtained markers were compared by study group, taking into account their standard deviations.

The results of such a study separately for each risk group are presented in Tables 28 and 29.

As in the case of the Russian women's population, the following rule was followed in the Tajik women's population. When prognostically significant values in group 6 or 7 exceeded the 95% confidence intervals in the other groups, the maximum value in the comparison groups was taken as the boundary of the prognostically significant range. among those in the comparison groups. If, on the contrary, the predictive value in group 6 or 7 was below the 95% confidence intervals in the other groups, the smallest value among the comparison groups was taken as the boundary of the predictive range.

Table 28. Borderline values and prognostically significant values for immunological parameters in women Tajik population for group 6

Informative indicators	Upper/ lower boundary for groups 1	Upper/ lower boundary for groups 2	Upper/ lower boundary for groups of 3	Prognostically significant range values in group 3
1	**2**	**3**	**4**	**5**
T-helpers (CD3+CD4+), %	max 33,2	min 33,2	max 31,4	> 33,2%
1	**2**	**3**	**4**	**5**
Cytotoxic T-lymphocytes	min 19,5	max 21,6	min 19,2	< 19,2%

ECT (CD3+CD56+),	max 1,7	min 3,5	max 2,2	> 2,2%
Natural killer cells	max 11,6	min 17,2	max 13,8	> 13,8%
B-lymphocytes (CD19+), %	max 13,6	min 14,2	max 14,2	> 14,2%
IgG, mg/ml	max	min	max	> 12.8 mg/ml

Note: grey indicates borderline prognostically significant value

As it follows from Table 46, prognostically significant values of markers of reproductive disorders were established for group 6, following the rule described above. As for the similar analysis for group 7, the results are shown in Table 27.

Table 29. Borderline values and prognostically significant values for immunological parameters in women Tajik population for group 7

Informative indicators	Upper/ lower boundary for groups 1	Upper/ lower boundary for groups 2	Upper/ lower boundary for groups of 3	Prognostically significant range values in group 3
IgG-antibodies to phospholipids,	max 9,0	max 8,2	min 10,6	> 9.0 units/ml
IgG-antibodies to β_2 -	max 7,8	max 8,0	min 10,2	> 8.0 units/ml
IgG-antibodies to prothrombin,	max 8,7	max 8,7	min 9,2	> 8.7 units/ml

Note: grey indicates borderline prognostically significant value

Thus, it was possible not only to establish the indicators that can serve as risk markers for reproductive health disorders in the population of Tajik women, but also to specify the ranges of their prognostically significant values for the formation of risk groups at the preclinical stage, while deviations in laboratory parameters are within the zone of reference values.

Summary to chapter 5

1. In the population of Russian women, immunological shifts associated with reproductive health disorders were registered in group 2 and included an increase in the number of lymphocytes with phenotypes CD3+CD4+, CD3+CD8+, CD3+CD56+, CD16+CD56+, CD19+, an increase in IgG levels, an increase in the blood content of autoantibodies to phospholipids and β - glycoprotein. $_{2}$
2. In the population of Tajik women, immunological shifts associated with reproductive health disorders were observed in group 5 and included an increase in the number of lymphocytes with CD3+CD4+, CD3+CD56+, CD16+CD56+, CD19+ phenotypes, as well as an increase in IgG levels and a drop in the number of CD3+CD8+ lymphocytes.
3. In the population of Tajik women, signs of antiphospholipid reactions associated with reproductive health disorders were observed in group 6 and included an increase in the level of IgG-autoantibodies to phospholipids, β_2 -glycoprotein and prothrombin.
4. The results of determining markers of possible reproductive health disorders (belonging to risk groups) in the studied populations of Russian and Tajik women are summarised and presented in Table 30:

Table 30. Markers of immunological shifts associated with with reproductive health problems

Studied populations	Marker is an indicator hormonal status	Value range marker
Russian population women, group 2	T-helper cells (CD3+CD4+)	> 35,7%
	Cytotoxic T-lymphocytes (CD3+CD8+)	> 20,2%
	EKT (CD3+CD56+)	> 4,2%
	Natural killer cells (CD16+CD56+)	> 14,6%
	B-lymphocytes (CD19+)	> 9,3%
	IgG	> 10.6 mg/ml
	IgG-antibodies to phospholipids	> 3.6 units/ml
	IgG-antibodies to β -glycoprotein$_2$	> 4.8 units/ml
Tajik Women's Population, group 6	T-helper cells (CD3+CD4+)	> 33,2%
	Cytotoxic T-lymphocytes (CD3+CD8+)	< 19,2%
	EKT (CD3+CD56+)	> 2,2%
	Natural killer cells (CD16+CD56+)	> 13,8%
	B-lymphocytes (CD19+)	> 14,2%
	IgG	> 12.8 mg/ml
Tajik Women's Population, group 7	Total IgG antibodies to	> 9.0 units/ml
	IgG-antibodies to β -glycoprotein$_2$	> 8.0 units/ml
	IgG-antibodies to prothrombin	> 8.7 units/ml

CHAPTER 6. PROGNOSTIC EFFICIENCY OF RISK MARKERS OF WOMEN'S REPRODUCTIVE HEALTH DISORDERS OF DIFFERENT POPULATIONS

6.1 Effectiveness of the system for determining the risk of violations Reproductive health of women in the Russian population

6.1.1 Development of integral markers of disorders Reproduction in women of the Russian population

In the previous sections of the study, it was shown that in the population of Russian women, in addition to women with preserved reproductive health, two categories of women (groups 2 and 3) with possible reproductive health disorders can be distinguished already at the preclinical stage, but characterised by different pathogenesis and, accordingly, different markers of such disorders. For group 2, 8 such markers were identified from immunological data, and for group 3, 7 markers were identified from hormonal status indicators. The objective of this section of the research is to try to develop, on this basis, integral markers for each risk group, which would take into account the contribution of each informative indicator to the overall system of predicting reproductive health disorders for each risk group.

To fulfil this task, first of all, it was determined with what frequency each of the markers was registered in each group of Russian women surveyed in order to clarify the role of individual markers in the overall testing system. The results of such a study for all study groups of women in the Russian population are presented in Table 31 and Figures 82-83.

Table 31: Frequency of occurrence of risk markers in study groups of women in the Russian population

Risk group markers		Result	Frequency of occurrence (people/%)			One way ANOVA	
			Group 1 n = 28	Group 2 n = 27	Group 3 n = 26	F	p
1		2	3	4	5	6	7
Group 2 risk markers	T-helper cells (CD3+CD4+) > 35.7%	+	7 / 25%	25 / 93%	9 / 35%	881,0	<0,001
		-	21 / 75%	2 / 7%	17 / 65%		
	Cytotoxic T-lymphocytes (CD3+CD8+) >20.2%	+	-	27 / 100%	-	881,0	<0,001
		-	28 / 100%	-	26 / 100%		
	EKT (CD3+CD56+) > 4.2%	+	-	25 / 93%	-	35,94	<0,001
		-	28 / 100%	2 / 7%	26 / 100%		
	Natural killer cells (CD16+ CD56+) > 14.6%	+	-	27 / 100%		881,0	<0,001
		-	28 / 100%	-	26 / 100%		
	B-lymphocytes (CD19+) > 9.3%	+	-	22 / 82%	-	115,0	<0,001
		-	28 / 100%	5 / 18%	26 / 100%		
	IgG > 10.6 mg/ml	+	6 / 22%	24 / 89%	5 / 20%	8,016	<0,001
		-	22 / 78%	3 / 11%	21 / 80%		
	IgG-antibodies to phospholipids > 3.6 units/ml	+	7 / 25%	25 / 93%	6 / 23%	46,88	<0,001
		-	21 / 75%	2 / 7%	20 / 77%		
	IgG-antibodies to β-glycoprotein	+	-	27 / 100%	-	447,4	<0,001
		-	28 / 100%	-	26 / 100%		
Group 3 risk	Luteinising hormone > 5.1 IU/L	+	2 / 8%	6 / 23%	25 / 97%	58,14	<0,001
		-	26 / 92%	21 / 77%	1 / 3%		
	Prolactin > 136 nmol/l	+	-	-	26 / 1007%	208,8	<0,001
		-	28 / 100%	27 / 100%	-		

	Estradiol > 237 pmol l	+	-	1 / 4%	26 / 100%	881,0	<0,001
		-	28 / 100%	26 / 96%	-		

Continuation of Table 31

1	2	3	4	5	6	7	8
Group 3 risk markers	Progesterone > 26.5 nmol/l	+	2 / 8%	3 / 12%	26 / 100%	287,8	<0,001
		-	26 / 92%	24 / 88%	-		
	Thyroid hormone > 1.6 mIU/l	+	3 / 11%	1 / 4%	24 / 93%	118,6	<0,001
		-	25 / 89%	26 / 96%	2 / 7%		
	Total thyroxine > 86.5 nmol/l	+	1 / 4%	1 / 4%	26 / 100%	881,0	<0,001
		-	27 / 96%	26 / 96%	-		
	Cortisol < 291 nmol/l	+	-	-	26 / 100%	304,0	<0,001
		-	28 / 100%	27 / 100%	-		

Note: n - number of women in the group; F - Fisher's criterion for the distribution of positive marker results in different groups; p - probability of differences in the distribution according to Fisher's criterion; grey colour indicates the reliability of differences at $p < 0.05$.

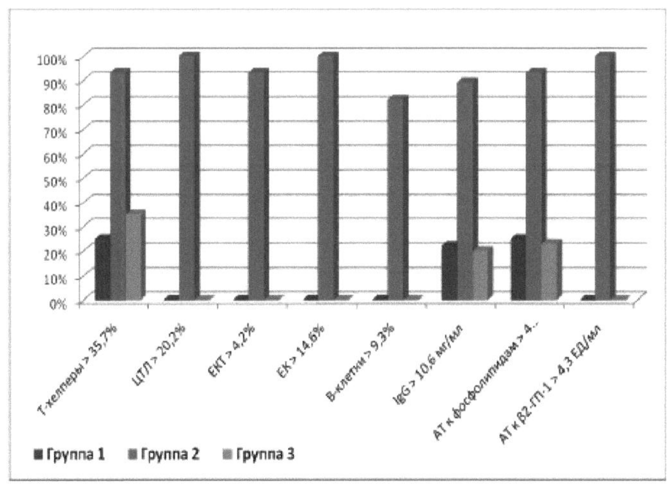

Figure 82. Frequency of individual markers of reproductive disorders associated with immunological shifts, in the study groups

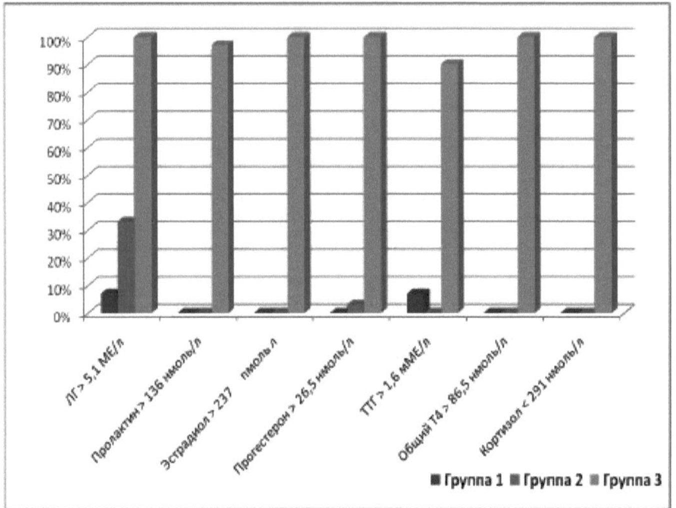

Figure 83. Frequency of occurrence of selected markers of reproductive disorders associated with hormonal shifts, in the study groups

The data shown in the table and figures clearly demonstrate that all selected indicators can fully correspond to the level of markers of the two categories of reproductive health disorders. This is evidenced by the reliability of the statistical evaluation of the data in each group, for which the ONE WAY ANOVA statistical method was used. The peculiarity of this method is that it reveals differences between frequency data even in cases where there is a single number of observations or even no observations in individual groups.

Thus, a total of 8 markers were selected to assess risk group 2 with predominant immunological shifts (Figure 82). All of these markers were noted in 22 people (82%) in group 2, 1 person in this group (4%) had 6 markers out of 8 and 4 people in group 2 had 5 markers out of 8. These data show that in isolated cases where a woman is found to have, for example, 5 or 6 markers out of 8, it is difficult to interpret the findings.

As for the occurrence of markers of hormonal shifts (Figure 83) characteristic of risk group 3, they are, as one would expect, clearly expressed in this group. In the other study groups, these markers are found in isolated cases. The only exception to this rule is a higher level of luteinising hormone, which is registered in about one fourth of women in risk group 2, which does not prevent these women from being classified as at risk for reproductive health disorders.

In addition, the results obtained both in the analysis of markers of risk group 2 and risk group 3 allow us to suggest that the diagnostic value of each of the markers is ambiguous; therefore, it would be desirable to obtain a different weight coefficient for each indicator and to develop the principle of integral assessment for predicting the risk of reproductive disorders in women of the Russian population, mainly of immunological and hormonal genesis.

In accordance with the put forward assumption, regression analysis was performed on all 8 traits of the risk group associated with immunological shifts, and a regression equation was obtained, presented as formula 2.

Formula 2

0.257*[CTL number] + 0.266*[EC number] + 0.122*[B-lf number] +

+ 0.107*[IgG level] + 0.209*[AT level to β_2 -GP]

In the process of obtaining the regression equation the statistical programme excluded 3 indicators (the number of T-helpers, the number of EKT and the level of antibodies to human phospholipids), and of the remaining 5 blood indicators the number of cytotoxic T-lymphocytes, the number of natural killer cells and the level of IgG-autoantibodies to β_2 -glycoproteins were the most informative, judging by the value of weight coefficients.

The obtained data have not only applied significance, but also allow us to draw a conclusion about some pathogenetic features of the development of reproductive disorders involving immune mechanisms, since they suggest that they are based on the cytotoxic potential of immune system cells, as well as elements of antiphospholipid reactions with disorders in the haemostasis system.

Then, in women of all studied groups, the data corresponding to 5 informative markers of group 2 were substituted into the regression equation. As a result, in each case we obtained an indicator, which we hereinafter refer to as the ***integral marker of reproductive impairment 1 (IMNR1)***.

Based on the obtained integral marker in each group, its 95% confidence intervals were determined and ROC curves were constructed with AUROC calculation as shown in Figure 84.

As it follows from the figure, determination of the integral marker on the basis of the linear regression equation makes it possible to bring the prognostic value of the test almost to the absolute value (AUROC = 1.0). A more detailed analysis using the standard deviations of the 95% confidence interval showed that the maximum deviation in the comparison groups was 11.5 and, therefore, values above 11.5 are a prognostically significant deviation of IMNR1.

In other words, using 5 immunological indicators and the proposed regression equation, we can calculate the value of the integral marker, which, with a value >11.5, allows us to assign a woman to a risk group for reproductive health disorders associated with immunological mechanisms.

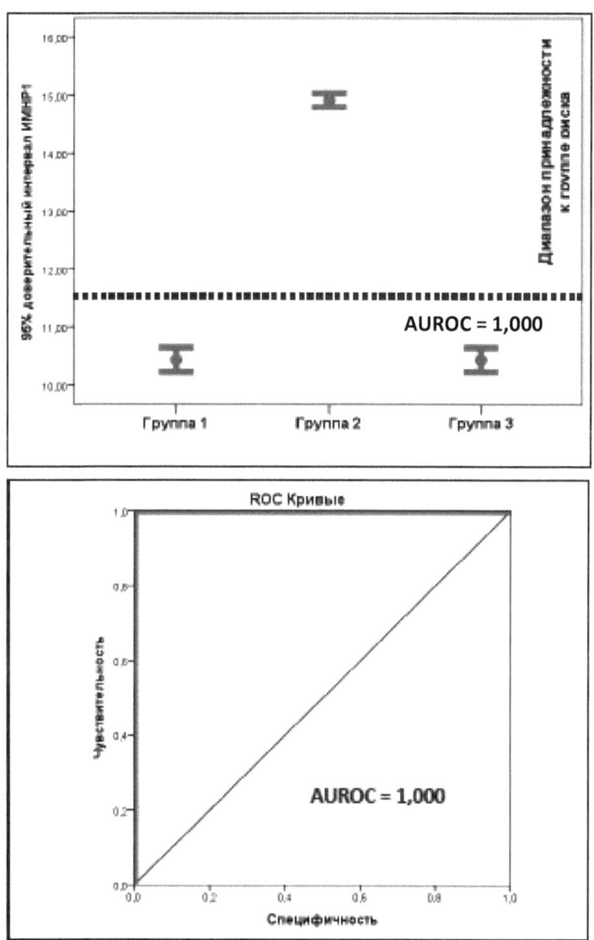

Figure 84. 95% confidence intervals of the integral marker of reproductive disorders 1 (IMNR1) due to immunological shifts in women of the Russian population and ROC curve of the predictive value of the test

(the dotted line indicates the boundary between the ranges of values prognostically significant values of IMNR and those in the comparison groups)

A similar study based on regression analysis was conducted for risk group 3. In this case, using 7 indicators of hormonal status, the regression equation presented in formula 3 was also obtained.

Formula 3

0.341*[prolactin] + 0.257*[estradiol] + 0.184*[total T4] -.

- 0.153*[cortisol].

In this case, three indicators - levels of luteinising hormone, progesterone, thyroid hormone - were excluded from the formula by the statistical programme, and the remaining 4 indicators were included in the regression equation, with prolactin (weight coefficient 0.341) and estradiol (weight coefficient 0.257) levels being the most informative.

The results of calculation of the integral marker in all observed women (*integral marker of reproductive disorders 2 - IMNR2*) followed by group determination of its 95% confidence interval and its corresponding AUROC are presented in Figure 85.

As can be seen in the figure, the determination of IMNR2 based on the linear regression equation yielded a diagnostic test whose predictive value, as in the case of IMNR1, was extremely high (AUROC = 0.996).

A detailed analysis of the standard deviations of the regression equations for the comparison groups (groups 1 and 2) showed that their maximum is 82. Consequently, if the values of IMNR2 are higher than 85, a woman at the prenosological stage can be reasonably attributed to the risk group for reproductive health disorders associated with hormonal shifts.

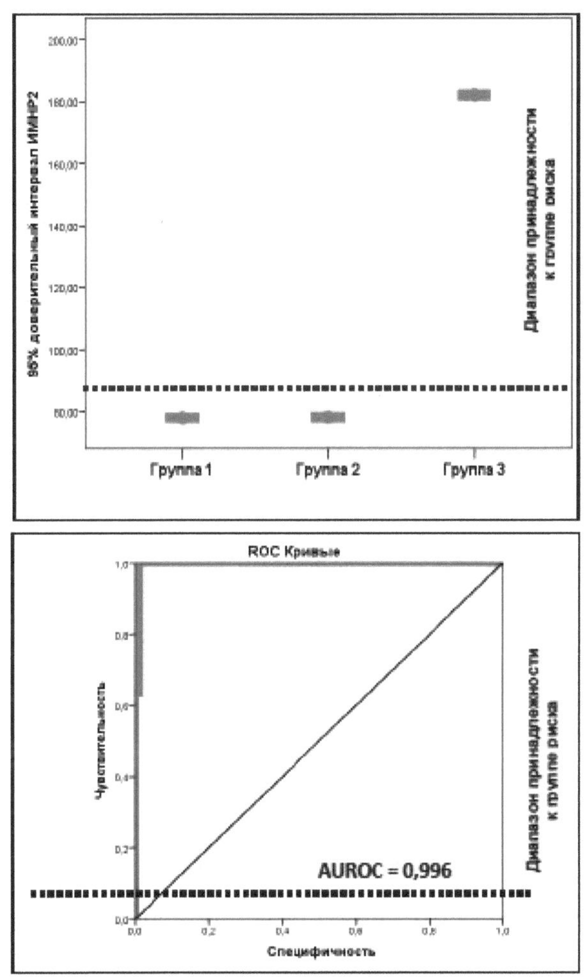

Figure 85. 95% confidence intervals of the integral marker of reproductive impairment 2 (IMNR2) due to hormones shifts in women in the Russian population and the ROC curve of the predictive value of the test

(the dotted line indicates the boundary between the ranges of values prognostically significant values of IMNR and those in the comparison groups)

Thus, for the Russian population of women, it was possible to develop two integral markers which, with almost absolute prognostic significance, allow us to assume reproductive disorders of various genesis in them.

6.1.2 Monitoring the effectiveness of integral markers in recognising reproductive health disorders in women in the Russian population

To control the effectiveness of the developed integral markers of reproductive disorders 1 and 2 in women of the Russian population, a group of 30 unmarried women was specially formed. These were recently married young women who had not given birth before the examination but were planning to become pregnant in the near future. These women with no obstetric history made up the study group number 4.

The aim of group 4 was to try to prognostically assess the state of reproductive health in these women using the integral markers of reproductive disorders (IMNR1 or IMNR2) developed by us, in order to confirm or not to confirm their effectiveness. For this purpose, all women in this group were followed up for a long term (3-year) follow-up of their fertility after laboratory examination. Four women who did not become pregnant during the following three years were subsequently excluded from the study, as this phenomenon may be based on disorders of not only female but also male reproductive health or a high degree of concordance between the genotypes of the couple.

Characteristics of informative laboratory parameters of this group of 26 women in terms of their compliance with the reference values for the Russian population included in IMNR1 and IMNR2, as well as the degree to which laboratory parameters fall within the ranges of prognostically significant values are presented in Table 32.

Table 32. Characterisation of comparison group 4 (unborn women in the Russian population) in terms of their compliance with reference values and the presence of risk markers

Risk group markers as components of IMNR1 and IMNR2	**Referenc e range values**	**Percentage of women with a value in the**	**Number/per centage of women with a risk**
Cytotoxic T cells (CD3+CD8+) > 20.2%	16,8 - 26,8	26 / 100%	2 / 8%
Natural killer cells (CD16+CD56+) > 14.6%	10,6 - 18,8	26 / 100%	2 / 8%
B-lymphocytes (CD19+) > 9.3%	5,4 - 13,6	26 / 100%	1 / 4%
IgG > 10.6 mg/ml	8,6 - 13,6	26 / 100%	7 / 27%
IgG-antibodies to β_2 - glycoprotein-1 > 4.3	2,0 - 7,2	26 / 100%	3 / 12%
Prolactin > 136 mIU/ml	121,0 - 224.2	26 / 100%	8 / 31%
Estradiol > 237 pmol/l	228,0 - 253,6	26 / 100%	14 / 54%
Total thyroxine > 86.5nmol/l	78,8 - 120,0	26 / 100%	3 / 12%
Cortisol < 291 nmol/L	214,3 - 341,9	26 / 100%	5 / 20%

As the table shows, all of the tested indicators for women in Group 4 are fully within the reference ranges. At the same time, between 1 and 14 of the women in group 4 may have indicators that are part of the IMNR1 and IMNR2 integral markers within the risk ranges for each indicator established in Chapters 4 and 5. It is difficult to assume that all randomly selected and clinically healthy women have reproductive health disorders, and the fact that their individual blood parameters fall within the ranges of prognostically significant values once again shows that each individual indicator, as well as their arbitrary aggregate, can hardly serve as criteria for predicting impaired reproductive functions. In this regard, special attention should be paid to the control of the effectiveness of such a prognosis, not by individual laboratory signs, but by integral markers of reproductive disorders.

For this purpose, both regression equations were calculated for each woman in group 4 to determine integral markers of reproductive health impairment 1 and 2 (IMNR1 and IMNR2). The raw data and the results of the calculations of both integral markers, taking into account the results of the follow-up obstetric and gynaecological follow-up of each of the 26 women over the next three years, are presented in full in Table 33

Table 33. Individual data and determination results IMNR1 and IMNR2 in women who have not given birth

No. n/a	**Input data and results of the IMNR calculation1 (prognostically significant range > 11.5)**	**Input data and results of the IMNR2 calculation (prognostically significant range > 85)**	**Obstetric 3 summer cathamnesis**
1	**2**	**3**	**4**
1.	0,257*16,7 + 0,266*12,6 + + 0,122*7,9 + 0,107*10,3 + + 0,209*6,2 = **11,04**	0,341*310,7 + 0,257*300,8 + + 0,184*83,4 - 0,153*309,0 = = **151,33**	One pregnancy not carried to term and one pregnancy resulting in the birth of a healthy childa
2.	0,257*17,0 + 0,266*12,6 + 0,122*6,0 + 0,107*9,5 + + 0,209*2,4 = **10,0**	0,341*139,0 + 0,257*232,0 + + 0,184*82,3 - 0,153*312,5 = = **74,36**	One pregnancy ended with a healthy baby being born

3.	0,257*17,7 + 0,266*11,6 + + 0,122*8,2 + 0,107*9,8 + + 0,209*7,0 = **10,17**	0,341*130,6 + 0,257*268,4 + + 0,184*84,7 - 0,153*310,0 = = **81,20**	One pregnancy ended with a healthy baby being born
4.	0,257*17,2 + 0,266*11,7 + + 0,122*5,0 + 0,107*10,5 + + 0,209*2,3 = **9,76**	0,341*127,6 + 0,257*259,6 + + 0,184*84,6 - 0,153*308,1 = = **78,38**	One pregnancy ended with a healthy baby being born
5.	0,257*17,3 + 0,266*13,2 + + 0,122*6,3 + 0,107*9,3 +	0,341*130,1 + 0,257*200,9 + + 0,184*125,7 - 0,153*210,6 =	Miscarriage of one pregnancy

Continued in Table 33

1	2	3	4
6.	0,257*24,8 + 0,266*16,8 + + 0,122*12,9 +0,107*11,7 +	0,341*138,7 + 0,257*231,3 + + 0,184*83,4 - 0,153*307,7 =	premature loss labour foetus
7.	0,257*17,7 + 0,266*10,4 + + 0,122*6,0 + 0,107*8,6 + [illegible]	0,341*130,1 + 0,257*230,0 + + 0,184*84,7 - 0,153*310,7 = [illegible]	Two pregnancies resulted in healthy babies
8.	0,257*18,5 + 0,266*11,9 + + 0,122*7,4 + 0,107*10,2 + + 0,209*2,4 =	0,341*130,0 + 0,257*249,5 + + 0,184*87,8 - 0,153*311,2 = = **77,0**	One pregnancy ended with a healthy baby being born
9.	0,257*16,5 + 0,266*13,5 + + 0,122*7,3 + 0,107*10,6 +	0,341*132,2 + 0,257*230,0 + + 0,184*85,3 - 0,153*308,2 =	One pregnancy ended with a healthy baby being born
10.	0,257*18,8 + 0,266*11,9 + + 0,122*7,2 + 0,107*10,8 +	0,341*131,3 + 0,257*258,0 + + 0,184*83,9 - 0,153*310,2 =	One pregnancy ended with a healthy baby being born
11.	0,257*17,0 + 0,266*11,2 + + 0,122*4,7 + 0,107*9,7 +	0,341*132,5 + 0,257*269,8 + + 0,184*89,9 - 0,153*309,0 =	One pregnancy ended with a healthy baby being born
12.	0,257*20,6 + 0,266*12,4+ + 0,122*5,3 + 0,107*7,9 +	0,341*138,0 + 0,257*241,5 + + 0,184*84,6 - 0,153*252,2 =	Miscarriage of one pregnancy

13 .	0,257*18,7 + 0,266*12,3 + + 0,122*6,1 + 0,107*10,1 +	0,341*139,0 + 0,257*219,0 + + 0,184*83,8 - 0,153*291,0 =	One pregnancy ended with a healthy baby being born
14 .	0,257*19,9 + 0,266*10,4 + + 0,122*6,3 + 0,107*9,5 +	0,341*129,6 + 0,257*280,3 + + 0,184*82,2 - 0,153*310,5 =	One pregnancy ended with a healthy baby being born
15 .	0,257*19,2 + 0,266*12,4 + + 0,122*5,5 + 0,107*10,3 +	0,341*131,1 + 0,257*270,0 + + 0,184*84,9 - 0,153*310,7 =	One pregnancy ended with a healthy baby being born
16 .	0,257*18,4 + 0,266*12,9 + + 0,122*7,0 + 0,107*9,8 +	0,341*138,4 + 0,257*271,5 + + 0,184*81,7 - 0,153*308,6 =	One pregnancy ended with a healthy baby being born

Continuation of Table 31

17 .	0,257*17,8 + 0,266*13,9 + + 0,122*7,8 + 0,107*11,1 + + 0,209*2,4 = **11,15**	0,341*139,3 + 0,257*274,0 + + 0,184*80,9 - 0,153*317,0 = = **84,31**	One pregnancy ended with a healthy baby being born
1	**2**	**3**	**4**
18 .	0,257*17,4 + 0,266*11,3 + + 0,122*8,3 + 0,107*8,8 +	0,341*131,6 + 0,257*227,0 + + 0,184*84,8 - 0,153*308,2 =	One pregnancy ended with a healthy baby being born
19 .	0,257*17,7 + 0,266*13,6 + + 0,122*7,2 + 0,107*9,4 +	0,341*131,0 + 0,257*270,3 + + 0,184*84,6 - 0,153*307,4 =	Two pregnancies ended up giving birth to healthy babies
20 .	0,257*18,1 + 0,266*15,2 + + 0,122*5,0 + 0,107*11,9 +	0,341*135,6 + 0,257*220,0 + + 0,184*85,6 - 0,153*309,9 =	One pregnancy ended with a healthy baby being born
21 .	0,257*17,8 + 0,266*10,6 + + 0,122*6,1 + 0,107*9,3 +	0,341*131,0 + 0,257*221,5 + + 0,184*85,7 - 0,153*290,2 =	One pregnancy ended with a healthy baby being born
22 .	0,257*18,5 + 0,266*11,2 + + 0,122*8,7 + 0,107*9,5 +	0,341*130,2 + 0,257*263,0 + + 0,184*84,8 - 0,153*312,3 =	One pregnancy ended with a healthy baby being born

23.	0,257*19,5 + 0,266*10,0 + + 0,122*6,3 + 0,107*9,5 +	0,341*320,0 + 0,257*301,5 + + 0,184*85,7 - 0,153*207,5 =	There is a history of non-pregnancy
24.	0,257*18,1 + 0,266*11,6 + + 0,122*6,6 + 0,107*11,1 +	0,341*131,4 + 0,257*218,7 + + 0,184*85,3 - 0,153*211,4 =	One pregnancy ended with a healthy baby being born
25.	0,257*18,2 + 0,266*12,4 + + 0,122*5,4 + 0,107*11,0 +	0,341*135,4 + 0,257*220,0 + + 0,184*84,9 - 0,153*314,4 =	One pregnancy ended with a healthy baby being born
26.	0,257*17,6 + 0,266*13,4 + + 0,122*4,8 + 0,107*9,1 +	0,341*125,8 + 0,257*210,0 + + 0,184*85,4 - 0,153*310,5 =	One pregnancy ended with a healthy baby being born

Note: red colour indicates an unfavourable deviation of the marker from the Indicators of women with preserved reproductive health

As the table shows, the long-term (three-year) follow-up of 26 non stinging women with subsequently developed pregnancies/pregnancies showed that in 21 cases the pregnancies occurred and resulted in the birth of a healthy child, and in two cases even two children. Four women experienced a miscarriage (in one case combined with a second pregnancy that ended safely), and one woman had a previous devre mented labour with the loss of a child.

Determination of the integral marker of reproductive disorders associated with predominant shifts in immune status (IMNR1) allowed us to assign a woman to the risk group in only one case (IMNR1>11.5). This woman developed preterm labour at 28 weeks, and the foetus could not be saved.

Four women with pregnancy failure had high values of IMNR2 (>85) associated with hormonal shifts. In other words, in these cases, IMNR2 values clearly indicated the possibility of hormone-mediated reproductive dysfunction, although the hormonal status indicators in this case were within the reference values.

Thus, the proposed integral markers of reproductive health disorders IMNR1 and IMNR2 for the population of Russian women can actually serve as criteria for selection of women into the risk group for reproductive health disorders of immunological and hormonal genesis, respectively.

6.1.3 Algorithm for conducting screening tests for predicting reproductive health disorders at the prenosological stage in women of the Russian population

The conducted studies based on testing the indicators of hormonal status, immune status, and signs of antiphospholipid reactions not exceeding the reference values were used as the basis for the development of a scheme for predicting possible reproductive health disorders in women in the Russian population (Figure 86).

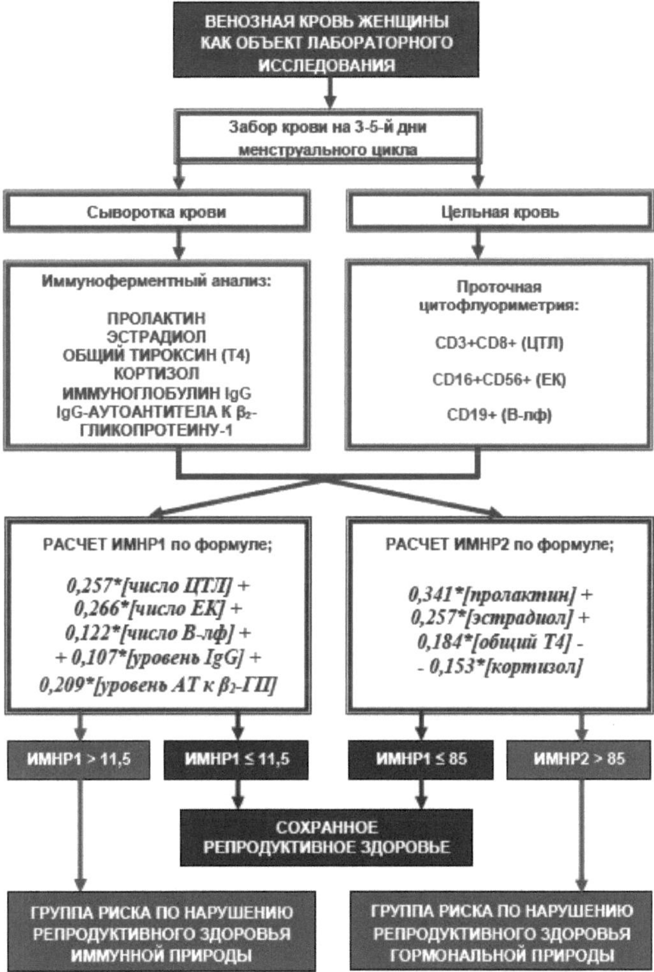

Fig. 86. Algorithm for predicting reproductive health disorders at the prenosological stage in women of the Russian population

As follows from the presented materials, the most relevant for the organisation of preventive measures to maintain reproductive health in young women in the absence of obstetric history and clinical signs of genital diseases (at the prenozological stage) is the prediction of the degree of risk of possible reproductive disorders.

From this point of view, our proposed algorithm for the examination of such women meets the requirements of modern health care and contributes to the solution of important medical and social problems.

It is recommended to examine women on the 3rd to 5th days of the menstrual cycle, as the examination scheme includes such hormones as oestradiol and prolactin, the determination of their levels is carried out exactly at these times.

Blood is collected as two samples in two tubes. One tube with EDTA to obtain a whole blood sample for phenotyping of lymphocytes (cytotoxic T-lymphocytes, natural killer cells, B-lymphocytes) by flow cytofluorimetry,

The second dry tube is intended for obtaining blood serum to determine in this biological material the levels of hormones (prolact tin, estradiol, total thyroxine, cortisol), immunoglobulins of IgG class, as well as IgG-autoantibodies to β_2 -glycoprotein I. The obtained quantitative laboratory data are substituted into the formulas for calculating IMNR1 and IMNR2.

A value of 11.5 is used as a criterion for assessing IMNR1. If a woman's IMNR1 is above this value, she is considered to be at risk for reproductive health problems. A detailed study of hormonal status and observation by an obstetrician-gynaecologist is recommended.

If IMNR1 is equal or lower than 11.5, the woman is considered to be conditionally healthy from the point of view of reproductive function. The same conclusion is made in cases when IMNR2 is equal to or lower than 85, because this value of this marker is the criterion value.

If the value of IMNR2 is above 85, the woman is also considered to be at risk of possible reproductive failure, but the recommendations for her examination, in addition to observation by an obstetrician-gynaecologist, include characteristic ristics of immune status - a wider range of phenotyping of lymphocytes, obtaining their functional characteristics, determining the levels of immunoglobulins, detecting autoantibodies to components of the thyroid gland, haemostasis system, phospholipids, tests for the presence of lupus anticoagulant in the blood, if necessary and if possible - immunogenetic studies about .

The tests outlined are not routine, yet they offer very specific new possibilities for predicting reproductive health disorders

6.2 Effectiveness of the system for determining the risk of violations Reproductive health of women in the Tajik population

6.2.1 Development of integral markers of disorders Reproduction in women of Tajik population

In the Tajik population of women, as defined in the previous sections of the study, the system of markers of reproductive health disorders within the established phenotypic and genotypic features differed significantly from those of Tajik women and also allowed for the identification of two categories of signs of reproductive disorders -

those associated with abnormalities in hormonal and immune status (group 6) or the development of antiphospholipid reactions (group 7).

For group 6, 12 markers from hormonal and immunological data were identified, and for group 7, 3 markers from signs of antiphospholipid reactions were identified. The task of this research section is to try to develop, on this basis, integral markers for each risk group (6 and 7), which would take into account the contribution of each informative indicator to the overall system of predicting reproductive health disorders for each risk group, as was done for the population of Russian women.

In order to fulfil this task, we first determined the frequency with which each marker was recorded in the groups of Tajik women surveyed in order to clarify the role of individual markers in the overall testing system. In addition, such an analysis would help to gain insight into whether it is sufficient to rely on single risk markers or whether it is advisable to proceed to the development of an integral marker. The results of such a study for all surveillance groups are summarised in Table 34 and Figures 87-88.

Table 33. Frequency of risk markers
in study groups of women in the Tajik population

Risk group markers		**Result**	**Frequency of occurrence (people/%)**			**One way ANOVA**	
			Group 1	**Group 2**	**Group 3**	**F**	**p**
1		**2**	**3**	**4**	**5**	**6**	**7**
Group 6 risk markers	Prolactin < 205 nmol/l	+	2 / 8%	28 / 93%	-	881,0	<0,001
		-	26 / 92%	-	28 / 100%		
	Estradiol < 245 pmol/l	+	2 / 8%	28 / 93%	-	881,0	<0,001
		-	26 / 92%	-	28 / 100%		
	Progesterone	+	2 / 8%	28 / 93%	3 / 11%		

	< 32.5 nmol/l	-	26 / 92%	-	25 / 89%	35,94	<0,001
1	**2**	**3**	**4**	**5**	**6**	**7**	**8**
Group	Autoantibodies to thyroglobulin > 2.9 ME/ml	+	1 / 4%	28 / 100%		881,0	<0,001
		-	27 / 96%	-	28 / 100%		

Continued in Table 33

	Autoantibodies to thyroperoxida	+	-	28 / 100%	1 / 4%	115,0	<0,001
		-	28 / 100%	-	27 / 96%		
	Cortisol > 254 nmol/l	+	2 / 8%	28 / 93%	-	8,016	<0,001
		-	26 / 92%	-	28 / 100%		
	T-helper cells (CD3+CD4+) > 33,2%	+	13 / 47%	27 / 94%	12 / 43%	46,88	<0,001
		-	15 / 53%	1 / 4%	16 / 57%		
	Cytotoxic T cells (CD3+CD8+)	+	4 /15%	20 / 72%	1 / 4%	447,4	<0,001
		-	24 / 85%	8 / 28%	27 / 92%		
	EKT (CD3+CD56+)	+	6 / 22%	28 / 100%	-	58,14	<0,001
		-	22 / 78%	-	28 / 100%		
	Natural killers (CD16+CD56+)	+	-	28 / 100%	-	208,8	<0,001
		-	28 / 100%	-	28 / 100%		
	B-lymphocytes (CD19+) >	+	3 / 11%	27 / 96%	3 / 11%	881,0	<0,001
		-	25 / 89%	1 / 4%	25 / 89%		
	IgG > 12.8 mg/ml	+	8 / 29%	28 / 100%	9 / 33%	287,8	<0,001
		-	20 / 71%	-	19 / 67%		
Group 7 risk markers	IgG-antibodies to phospholipids > 9 units/ml	+	-	-	27 / 96%	118,6	<0,001
		-	28 / 100%	28 / 100%	1 / 4%		
	IgG-antibodies to β-glycoprotein-1_2	+	1 / 4%	1 / 4%	28 / 100%	881,0	<0,001
		-	27 / 96%	27 / 96%	-		
		+	-	-	28 / 100%		

	IgG-antibodies to	-	28 / 100%	28 / 100%	-	304,0	<0,001

Note: n - number of women in the group; F - Fisher's criterion for the distribution of positive marker results in different groups; p - probability of differences in the distribution according to Fisher's criterion; grey colour indicates the reliability of differences at $p < 0.05$.

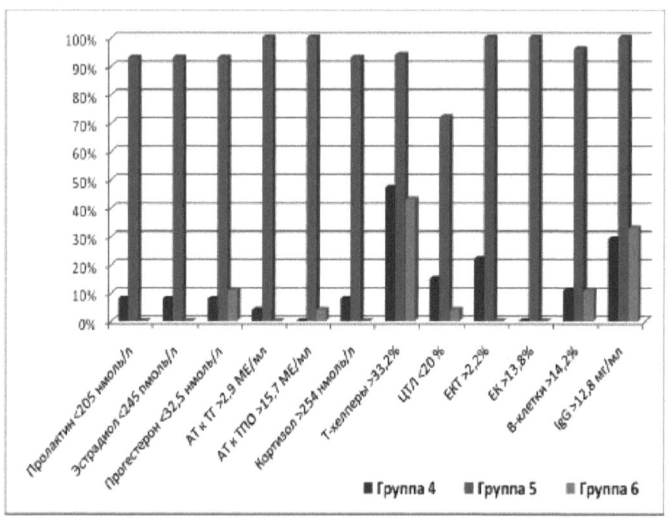

Figure 87. Frequency of occurrence of individual markers of reproductive disorders associated with hormonal and immunological shifts in the study groups of the Tajik population

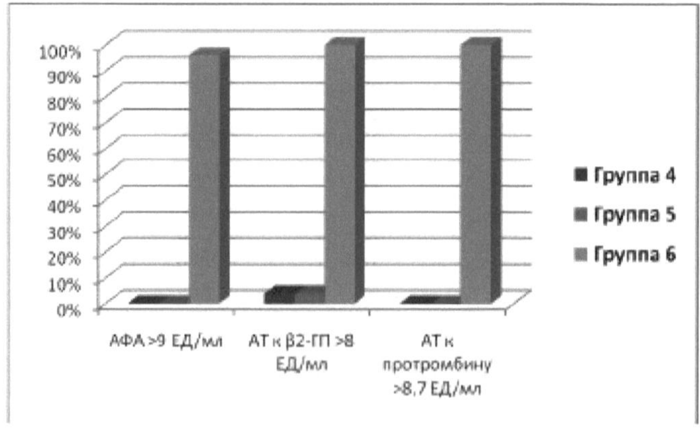

Figure 88. Frequency of occurrence of selected markers of reproductive disorders associated with antiphospholipid reactions, in the Tajik population study groups

The data presented in the table and figures fully confirm the effectiveness of markers of reproductive disorders associated both with hormonal and immunological abnormalities and with the development of antiphospho lipid reactions in a differentiated approach to their establishment.

Thus, markers of risk group 6 in the population of Tajik women are significantly higher in frequency of occurrence in this group and in no case show a value below 70%. In all other groups, the frequency of occurrence of these markers, as a rule, is in the range of 1-8%, although in some cases reaching 24-47%.

The few markers in risk group 7 are even more effective in recognising whether women belong to this group. In group 7 itself, the frequency of occurrence of these markers is between 93% and 100%, while in the other groups it does not exceed 4%.

At the same time, the occurrence of markers of risk groups in groups of healthy women, sometimes even significant, shows the target difference for a more accurate assessment of reproductive health disorders. By analogy with the population of Russian women, it was decided to use regression analysis to develop integral markers of reproductive disorders.

Regression analysis based on all 12 markers associated with hormonal and immunological signs of reproductive health disorders (risk group 6) yielded a regression equation (formula 4) that included only 2 immunological indicators out of 12:

Formula 4

-9.049 + 0.537*[EC count] - 0.208*[B-lymphocyte count]

As follows from the equation, the factors determining hormonal shifts were completely removed from its composition, despite the fact that all of them showed reliable differences between women in the risk group 6. This does not mean that these factors do not participate in the formation of reproductive health disorders in this group, they simply cannot be reliable markers of these disorders.

As for the two immunological markers included in the regression equation - the number of natural killer cells and the number of B-lymphocytes - they formed the so-called integral marker of reproductive disorders, which in the context of these studies we labelled as IMNR3.

To confirm the sufficiency and degree of prognostic significance of IMNR3, we further analysed the values of its 95% confidence intervals and ROC-curve with calculation of the area under the curve - AUROC. The results of such statistical analysis are presented in Figure 89.

The obtained graphs reflect the totality of all individual data in women of the Tajik population belonging to different study groups and show that the obtained regression equation and the immunological indices included in it fully characterise a woman's belonging to the risk group 6.

Detailed analysis using standard deviations of 95% confidence intervals showed that the maximum deviation in the comparison groups in Tajik women was 14.0 and, therefore, values above 14 were prognostically significant deviations of IMNR3. As for the prognostic significance of this test, it was close to absolute, judging by the AUROC value, as it was equal to 1.0.

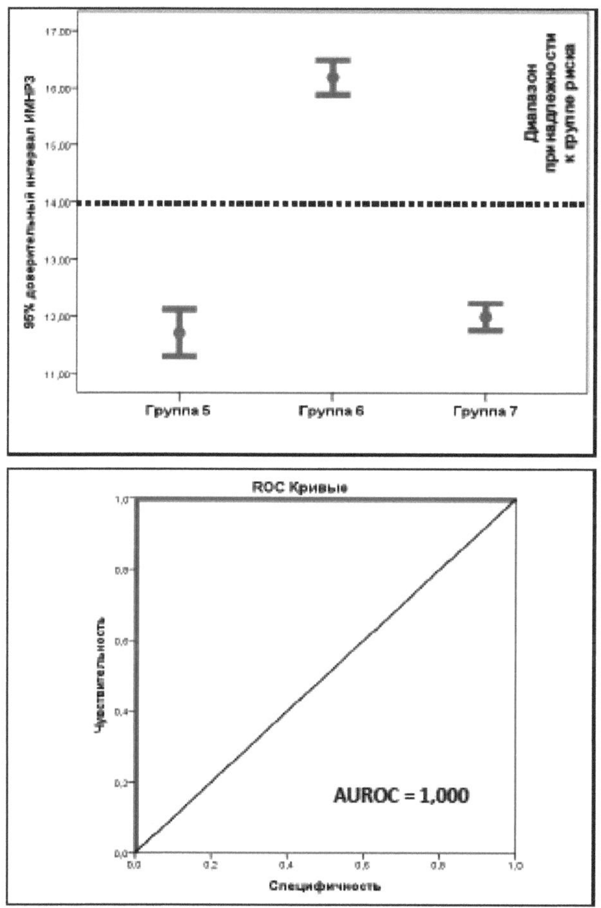

Figure 89. 95% confidence intervals of the integral marker of women in the Tajik population with reproductive health disorders due to immunological shifts (IMNR3) and the ROC curve of the predictive value of the test

(the dotted line indicates the boundary between the ranges of values prognostically significant values of IMNR and those in the comparison groups)

AUROC = 1,000

Regression analysis was also performed for risk group 7 on the basis of the characteristic for this group increase in the values of IgG-autoantibodies to human phospholipids (HPA), β_2 -glycoproteins, prothrombin. The obtained regression equation had the form of formula 5.

Formula 5

$$\boldsymbol{2.179 + 0.288*[APA] + 0.453*[AT\ to\ \beta\ \text{-}GP]_2}$$

This regression equation included only two indicators out of three, because the level of IgG autoantibodies to prothrombin did not participate in the formation of the integral marker of reproductive disorders (IMNR4), as it was excluded by the statistical programme.

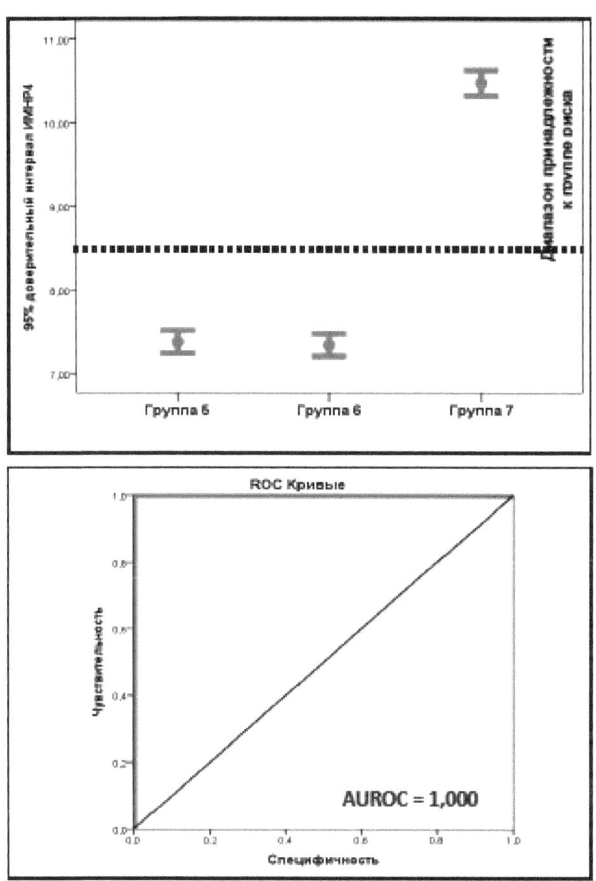

Figure 90. 95% confidence intervals of the integral marker of women in the Tajik population with antiphospholipid reaction-type reproductive disorders (IMNR4) and the ROC curve of the predictive value of the test
(the dotted line indicates the boundary between the ranges of values prognostically significant values of IMNR and those in the comparison groups)

The individual values of each woman who participated in the study were then substituted into the regression equation. The graphs for analysing the prognostically significant range of IMNR4 values based on 95% confidence intervals and the actual prognostic significance of the test based on the ROC curve are shown in Figure 90.

As follows from the graphs, the integral marker of reproductive disorders in group 7 (IMNR4), as well as in all other cases, allowed to determine with almost absolute clarity (AUROC = 1.0) the belonging of women to this group.

A detailed analysis using standard deviations of the 95% confidence interval showed that the maximum deviation in the comparison groups was 8.5 and, therefore, values higher than 8.5 are prognostically significant deviations of IMNR4 in determining the risk of reproductive dysfunctions.

Thus, for the Tajik population of women it was possible, as well as for the Russian population, to develop two integral markers that differ in principle from those in the Russian population and with almost absolute prognostic significance allow us to assume reproductive disorders of various genesis in Tajik women.

6.2.2 Monitoring the effectiveness of integral markers in recognising reproductive health disorders in women of the Tajik population

To further confirm how effectively the integral indicators developed in this section of the study, IMNR3 and IMNR4, can be applied in medical practice, they were tested on a specially selected group of 32 unborn Tajik women (group 8) who, as in the Russian population, were followed up by an obstetrician-gynaecologist for the next 3 years. This cohort was composed of young women planning pregnancy. However, 3 women did not become pregnant during the first year of follow-up and were referred for further evaluation and excluded from the cohort, while the remaining women were followed up.

Characteristics of informative laboratory indicators of the group of 8 out of 29 women in terms of their compliance with the reference values of indicators for the Tajik population included in the IMNR3 and IMNR4, as well as the degree to which their laboratory indicators fall within the ranges of prognostically significant values are presented in Table 35.

Table 35. Characteristics of the comparison group 8 (non-pregnant women of Tajik population) in terms of their compliance with reference values and presence of risk markers

Risk group markers as components of IMNR1 and IMNR2	Reference range values	Percentage of women with a value	Percentage of women with a risk
Natural killer cells (CD16+CD56+) >	8,7 - 20,1	29 / 100%	2 / 7%
B-lymphocytes (CD19+) > 14.2%	6,8 - 18,6	29 / 100%	4 / 14%
IgG antibodies to phospholipids	5,7 - 11,9	29 / 100%	-
IgG-antibodies to β_2 - glycoprotein-1 > 8	6,1 - 11,6	29 / 100%	3 / 10%

As follows from the table, all tested indicators of women in Group 8 are fully within the reference ranges. At the same time, up to 14% of women in this group show positive results for individual risk markers that are part of the integral markers of IMNR1 and IMNR2, but are not combined with each other. In this regard, special attention should be paid to monitoring the effectiveness of reproductive health disorders prognosis in this group, but not by individual laboratory signs, but by integral markers of reproductive disorders.

Table 36 presents a system for calculating individual values of each integral marker of reproductive disorders (IMNR3 and IMNR4) for each of the 29 unborn women in group 8 of the Tajik population, and compares these individual values with catamnestic data obtained from follow-up of these women for 3 subsequent years. Comparison of the results of IMNR calculation and obstetric catamnesis is aimed at confirming or not confirming the effectiveness of the proposed methodology.

Table 36. Individual data and results of determination of integral markers of reproductive disorders in unborn women of Tajik population

No. n/a	Baseline data and results of IMNR1 calculation (prognostically	Baseline data and results of IMNR2 calculation (prognostically	Obstetrical 3-summer cathamnesis
1	2	3	4
1.	-9,049 + 0,537*10,9 - 0,208*12,2 = **12,4**	2,179 + 0,288*6,3 + 0,453*7,2 = **7,3**	One pregnancy ended with a healthy baby being born
2.	-9,049 + 0,537*9,8 - 0,208*14,0 = **11,4**	2,179 + 0,288*6,8 + 0,453*7,2 = **7,4**	One pregnancy ended with a healthy baby being born
3.	-9,049 + 0,537*15,1 - 0,208*13,2 = **14,4**	2,179 + 0,288*6,4 + 0,453*7,1 = **7,2**	There has been a history of non-pregnancy
4.	-9,049 + 0,537*10,2 - 0,208*11,8 = **12,1**	2,179 + 0,288*6,4 + 0,453*7,3 = **7,3**	Two pregnancies ended up giving birth to healthy babies

Continuation of table 36

5.	-9,049 + 0,537*10,5 - 0,208*10,6 = **12,5**	2,179 + 0,288*6,8 + 0,453*7,4 = **7,5**	One pregnancy ended with a healthy baby being born
6.	-9,049 + 0,537*11,1 - 0,208*13,7 = **12,2**	2,179 + 0,288*7,3 + 0,453*7,6 = **7,7**	One pregnancy ended with a healthy baby being born
1	**2**	**3**	**4**
7.	-9,049 + 0,537*9,6 - 0,208*12,7 = **11,6**	2,179 + 0,288*5,8 + 0,453*7,6 = 7,**3**	One pregnancy ended with a healthy baby being born
8.	-9,049 + 0,537*10,4 - 0,208*14,0 = **11,7**	2,179 + 0,288*6,7 + 0,453*6,9 = **7,2**	One pregnancy ended with a healthy baby being born
9.	-9,049 + 0,537*10,7 - 0,208*11,1 = **12,5**	2,179 + 0,288*8,6 + 0,453*9,2 = **8,8**	One pregnancy ended in a premature delivery of the surviving baby
10.	-9,049 + 0,537*9,9 - 0,208*11,2 = **12,0**	2,179 + 0,288*7,2 + 0,453*7,4 = 7,**6**	One pregnancy ended with a healthy baby being born
11.	-9,049 + 0,537*15,3 - 0,208*12,4 = **14,7**	2,179 + 0,288*8,3 + 0,453*6,5 = **7,5**	There has been a history of non-pregnancy
12.	-9,049 + 0,537*10,3 - 0,208*11,9 = **12,1**	2,179 + 0,288*6,4 + 0,453*7,1 = **7,2**	One pregnancy ended with a healthy baby being born
13.	-9,049 + 0,537*10,5 - 0,208*13,7 = **11,8**	2,179 + 0,288*7,0 + 0,453*6,7 = **7,2**	One pregnancy ended with a healthy baby being born
14.	-9,049 + 0,537*9,7 - 0,208*16,1 = **10,9**	2,179 + 0,288*6,1 + 0,453*7,1 = 7,**2**	Two pregnancies ended up giving birth to healthy babies
15.	-9,049 + 0,537*10,4 - 0,208*12,5 = **12,0**	2,179 + 0,288*6,5 + 0,453*7,0 = **7,2**	One pregnancy ended with a healthy baby being born

Continuation of table 36

16.	-9,049 + 0,537*10,5 - 0,208*14,3 = **11,7**	2,179 + 0,288*6,2 + 0,453*6,9 = **7,1**	One pregnancy ended with a healthy baby being born
17.	-9,049 + 0,537*10,8 - 0,208*11,4 = **12,5**	2,179 + 0,288*6,9 + 0,453*6,6 = **7,2**	One pregnancy ended with a healthy baby being born
18.	-9,049 + 0,537*9,0 - 0,208*13,5 = **11,1**	2,179 + 0,288*6,1 + 0,453*7,9 = **7,5**	One pregnancy ended with a healthy baby being born
1	**2**	**3**	**4**
19.	-9,049 + 0,537*10,9 - 0,208*15,8 = **11,6**	2,179 + 0,288*6,1 + 0,453*8,0 = **7,6**	Two pregnancies ended up giving birth to healthy babies
20.	-9,049 + 0,537*9,9 - 0,208*9,0 = **12,5**	2,179 + 0,288*6,2 + 0,453*8,1 = **7,6**	Two pregnancies ended up giving birth to healthy babies
21.	-9,049 + 0,537*9,8 - 0,208*8,4 = **12,6**	2,179 + 0,288*6,3 + 0,453*8,0 = **7,6**	One pregnancy ended with a healthy baby being born
22.	-9,049 + 0,537*10,5 - 0,208*7,9 = **13,0**	2,179 + 0,288*6,6 + 0,453*5,6 = **6,6**	One pregnancy ended with a healthy baby being born
23.	-9,049 + 0,537*10,9 - 0,208*8,7 = **13,1**	2,179 + 0,288*7,0 + 0,453*7,1 = **7,4**	One pregnancy ended with a healthy baby being born
24.	-9,049 + 0,537*10,2 - 0,208*8,1 = **12,8**	2,179 + 0,288*6,5 + 0,453*6,2 = **6,9**	One pregnancy ended with a healthy baby being born
25.	-9,049 + 0,537*10,8 - 0,208*8,8 = **13,0**	2,179 + 0,288*9,0 + 0,453*8,6 = **8,7**	There is a history of non-pregnancy
26.	-9,049 + 0,537*9,9 - 0,208*15,0 = **11,2**	2,179 + 0,288*7,3 + 0,453*6,9 = **7,4**	One pregnancy ended with a healthy baby being born

27.	-9,049 + 0,537*10,5 - 0,208*11,9 = **12,2**	2,179 + 0,288*6,4 + 0,453*6,6 = **7,0**	One pregnancy ended with a healthy baby being born
28.	-9,049 + 0,537*9,8 - 0,208*9,5 = **12,3**	2,179 + 0,288*6,9 + 0,453*8,5 = **8,0**	Two pregnancies ended up giving birth to healthy babies
29.	-9,049 + 0,537*10,8 - 0,208*10,9 = **12,6**	2,179 + 0,288*6,9 + 0,453*7,5 = 7,6	Two pregnancies ended up giving birth to healthy babies

Note: red colour indicates an unfavourable deviation of the marker from the indicators of women with preserved reproductive health

As follows from the table, 25 women in the Tajik population, who had not had pregnancies before the study, developed pregnancies (and in 6 cases even 2) within the next 3 years, which resulted in the birth of healthy children. At the same time, none of the women with preserved reproductive function had values of IMNR3 > 14.0 and/or IMNR4 > 8.5, which are characteristic of reproductive disorders.

Four women in the Tajik population had reproductive health disorders. In three cases, it was manifested by non-pregnancy, which coincided with relatively high values of IMNR3 (14.4 and 14.7) and IMNR4 (8.7), and in one case the pregnancy ended in preterm labour with IMNR4 = 8.8.

Thus, in the population of Tajik women, the use of the integral markers IMNR3 and IMNR4, developed by us, made it possible in principle to determine whether a woman belongs to a risk group for reproductive health disorders at the prenosological stage. Depending on which of these two indicators is in the range of values characteristic of the development of reproductive disorders, it is possible to assume whether these disorders are associated with hormonal and immunological shifts (IMNR3) or with the presence of signs of antiphospholipid reactions in a woman (IMNR4).

6.2.3 Algorithm of screening tests for predicting reproductive health disorders at the prenosological stage in women of Tajik population

Taking into account the effectiveness of the integral markers IMNR3 and IMNR4 in predicting the possibility of reproductive disorders in women of the Tajik population, we proposed an algorithm for conducting research in the form of a scheme of laboratory screening for the determination of these markers.

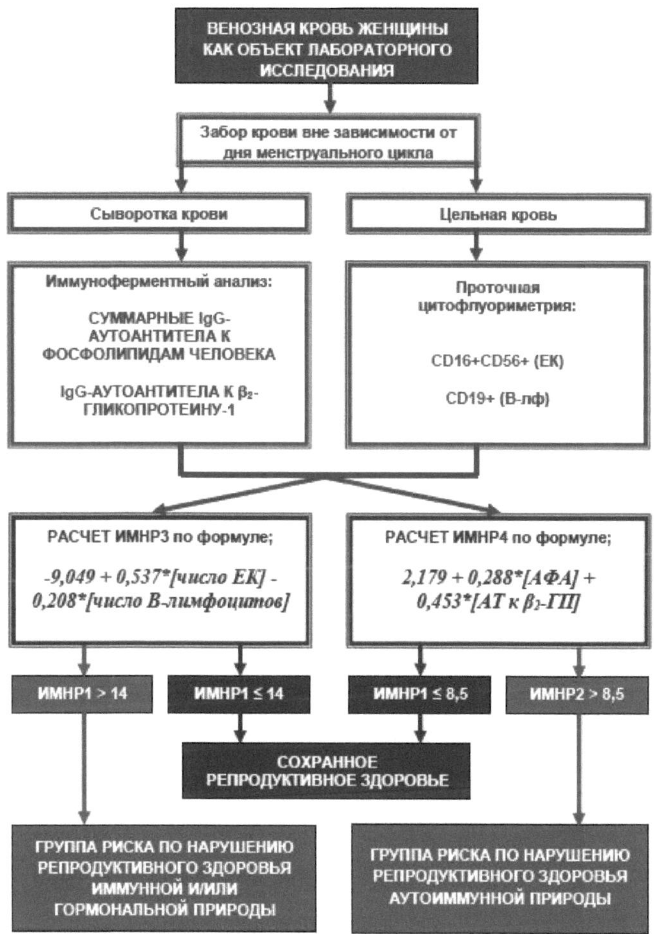

Fig. 91. Algorithm for predicting reproductive health disorders at the prenosological stage in women of the Tajik population

The recommended procedure for conducting studies based on testing the immunophenotypic characteristics of two categories of lymphocytes and the levels of two types of IgG autoantibodies, which are signs of anti- phospho lipid reactions but do not exceed reference values, is reflected in the scheme of Figure 90 for predicting possible reproductive health disorders in women in the Tajik population.

The algorithm for conducting research to predict reproductive health disorders in women of the Tajik population is very similar to the algorithm developed for women of the Russian population, although there are differences in the content of the research. These differences are due to differences in the formulas for calculating IMNR1 and IMNR2.

Firstly, laboratory testing to determine integral markers in the Tajik population does not need to be performed according to the menstrual cycle, as hormones in general and sex hormones in particular are not included in the examination scheme.

As already noted, the formulas for calculating IMNR3 and IMNR4 are unique and do not correspond to those for Russian women.

Finally, the quantitative way of assessing both integral markers is different. The criterion for determining whether a woman belongs to the risk group according to the value of IMNR3 lies in the area of values >14. In this case, the woman should be under the supervision of an obstetrician-gynaecologist and should undergo a laboratory study with detailed characterisation of hormonal and immune status.

In the case of IMNR4, values suggesting the possibility of reproductive health impairment are in the range of >8.5. Such women need, first of all, to exclude antiphospholipid reactions in them.

According to our data, values of IMNR3 and IMNR4 below the criterion values are favourable and indicate preservation of reproductive functions in women.

Summary to chapter 6

1. In the population of Russian women, reproductive disorders associated with immunological shifts can be identified and predicted at the prenosological stage using the newly developed integral marker IMNR1, calculated using the following formula: 0.257*[number of CTLs] + 0.266*[number of ECs] + 0.122*[number of B-lf] + 0.107*[IgG level] + 0.209*[AT level to β_2 -GP]. The presence of reproductive health disorders is evidenced by the value of IMNR1 > 11.5.
2. In the population of Russian women, reproductive disorders associated with hormonal shifts can be identified and predicted at the prenosological stage using the newly developed botan integrated marker IMNR2, calculated using the following formula: 0.341*[prolactin] + 0.257*[estradiol] + 0.184*[total T4] - 0.153*[cortisol]. The presence of reproductive health disorders is indicated by the value of IMNR2 > 85.
3. In the population of Tajik women, reproductive disorders associated with hormonal and immunological shifts can be identified and predicted at the prenosological stage using the newly developed integral marker IMNR3, calculated using the following formula: -9.049 + 0.537*[number of EC] - 0.208*[number of B-lymphocytes]. The presence of

reproductive health disorders is indicated by the value of IMNR3 > 14.

4. In the population of Tajik women, reproductive disorders associated with the development of antiphospholipid reactions can be identified and predicted at the prenosological stage using the newly developed integral marker IMNR4, calculated by the following formula: 2.179+0.288*[AFA] + 0.453*[AT to β_2 -GP]. The presence of reproductive health disorders is evidenced by the value of IMNR4 > 8.5.

CONCLUSION AND DISCUSSION

The following data covered in the domestic and foreign literature served as prerequisites for the research:

- The protection of women's reproductive health is one of the most important medical and social problems, without which neither economic nor social development of the state is possible [7, 8, 34, 74, 208].

- Both the physiological indicators of reproductive health and the nature of disorders of the latter depend on the climatic, geographical and environmental conditions in which a woman lives, on her ethnicity - [81, 101, 154].

-. The study of the role of immunogenetic factors in reproductive disorders is promising for predicting reproductive disorders and combating infertility - [11, 31, 57, 97].

- The importance of hormonal status in the formation of reproductive health is beyond doubt - [15, 40, 46, 28].

- Reproductive immunology, on the one hand, requires in-depth deciphering of immunological mechanisms and, on the other hand, needs reliable markers of immunopathological conditions associated with reproductive disorders - [57, 177].

- The development of autoimmune pathology contributes to hormonal shifts, formation of antiphospholipid reactions and leads to reproductive disorders in women [36, 114, 205].

- Causes and conditions of reproductive health disorders are closely related and are realised, as a rule, in complex combinations with each other - [53, 92, 99, 108].

- The example of antiphospholipid syndrome shows the prospect of developing scales for quantitative risk assessment of reproductive health disorders - [130, 28].

- The presence of clinical manifestations of genital lesions in women, as well as significant laboratory shifts associated with reproductive health disorders, contribute to the detection of the latter, but the issues of their prediction at the prenozological stage remain poorly understood and hinder their prevention in different ethnic groups - [152, 28].

Given these prerequisites, the aim of the study was to test a cluster-population approach to assessing the risk of reproductive health disorders in women of fertile age in the Russian and Tajik populations and to develop quantitative criteria for such assessment at the prenosological stage.

To realise this goal, a group of 1,025 clinically healthy women was selected, of whom 515 lived in Russia and 510 in the Republic of Tajikistan. All women under observation were in the fertile age range from 20 to 44 years, their average age was 28.1± 0.7 years. The population of Russian women included members of the Eastern Slavic ethnic group of Caucasoid race living in the Lipetsk region in a moderately continental climate. The population of Tajik women contained representatives of the Pamir-Fergana race of the Central Asian interfluve, the easternmost subrace of the Caucasoid race, living in Faizabad, a typical mountainous country with a subtropical sharply continental climate.

At the first stage, venous blood was collected from all 1025 women for HLA typing by molecular genetic analysis and to determine the range of normal values of hormonal and immune status indicators, the presence of autoantibodies and other signs of antiphospholipid reactions in each population. All examined women were clinically healthy at the time of the study.

For further research, women were additionally selected in accordance with the developed criteria for inclusion in the study and exclusion from the study. The main selection criterion was the absence of complaints of genitourinary tract diseases or their presence in the history, as well as the compliance of women's basic laboratory parameters with newly established population physiological norms.

Next, women from both populations underwent detailed laboratory examination for hormonal status (blood levels of follicle stimulating hormone, luteinising hormone, prolactin, estrogen, progesterone, testosterone, dihydroepiandrosterone, 17-OH-progesterone, thyro trope hormone, total triiodothyronine, total thyroxinea, cortisol), immune status (proportion of T-lymphocytes, T-helper cells, cytotoxic T-cells, ECT, natural killer cells, B-lymphocytes, levels of IgM, IgG, IgA), presence of autoimmune component (blood content of IgG-autoantibodies to thyroglobulin, thyroperoxidase, total phospholipids, β2-glycoprotein-1, annexin V, prothrombin, lupus anticoagulant).

Laboratory studies were performed using: molecular genetic analysis (PCR) method for typing allelic variants of HLA class II genes (DRB1, DQA1, DQB1 loci); indirect enzyme immunoassay method for determination of hormones, immunoglobulins, autoantibodies in blood serum; flow cytofluorimetry method for phenotyping of lymphocytes in whole blood; rapid Lupus test and lebetox test for detection of lupus anticoagulant in plasma.

Statistical processing of data was carried out on the basis of SPSS programmes and included discriminant statistics, discriminant, cluster, regression, single factor analysis of variance, calculation of 95% confidence intervals, construction of ROC curves.

The first objective of the study was to clarify physiological norms and identify population characteristics in women of fertile age in the Russian and Tajik populations, taking into account immunogenetic traits, hormonal and immune status data.

Using interactive **OLAP-cube** data analysis, reference ranges were obtained, and it was found that, in general, the range of variation in the reference values of the indicators in our study was somewhat narrower than indicated in the literature, which can be explained by the limitations of the female population.

In the population of Russian women, the reference values for blood androgens and thyroid hormones were slightly lower than generally accepted values, while in the population of Tajik women, on the contrary, the level of androgens in the blood was higher, and the content of thyroid hormones, except for total triiodothyronine, corresponded to generally accepted standards.

The deviations of the reference values of immune status indicators from the standard range were not very significant. In the Russian population of women, the percentages of T-helper cells, EKT, natural killer cells, and IgM levels were slightly higher, with a narrower range of variation. In the Tajik population, the most significant deviation in favour of an increase was given only by the proportion of T-helpers in the blood.

The reference values of the autoimmune component in both the population of Russian women and Tajik women were slightly higher than those shown in the recommendations of other authors, with the only difference being that Russian women had higher levels of autoantibodies to thyroid components and prothrombin, while Tajik women showed an increase in the levels of all autoantibodies tested.

Based on a refined normative interval with one standard deviation from the mean values, study groups were selected in each population whose laboratory values were within the reference values for more than 80% of the tests but had differences in obstetric history.

The following groups were formed according to obstetric history in each population of women of fertile age:

1) women who gave birth and whose pregnancy/pregnancies ended in the delivery of healthy children at term (control group with preserved reproductive function) - 28 people each in both the Russian and Tajik populations;

2) women who have given birth and have a history of pregnancy/pregnancy that ended in premature delivery, foetal failure, stillbirth (risk group with reproductive disorders) - 53 people in the Russian population and 57 people in the Tajik population;

3) unborn women planning pregnancy and intended for observation by an obstetrician-gynaecologist during the next three years after laboratory examination (a group for testing the methods of predicting the risk of reproductive disorders proposed in this work) - 26 people in the Russian population and 29 people in the Tajik population.

Further, population differences in the above groups were determined by a set of hormonal, immune traits, presence of autoimmune component, and immunogenetic features.

As the data obtained showed, there were significant differences in hormonal status between the populations of Russian and Tajik women, which extended, first of all, to the level of follicle-stimulating hormone, which was significantly higher in Russian women. In addition, significant differences were noted for the levels of progesterone, 17-OH-progesterone, dihydroepiandogen sulphate, and thyroid hormone, which were higher in Tajik women.

These data in themselves are of undoubted interest, since we have not found such comparative studies for these populations in the available literature. At the same time, D.A. Hojamuradova and T.A. Nazarenko [93] in their study emphasised a more frequent variant of hormonal function reduction in women of the Republic of Tajikistan than hyperhormonal shifts.

As a result of determining possible differences between the immune status of women of different populations, it was found that the blood content of T-lymphocytes, T-helpers, and IgM levels did not differ significantly. The relative number of cytotoxic T-lymphocytes, B-cells, and IgG levels were higher in the Tajik women population, while the number of EKT and natural killer cells and IgA levels deviated quite significantly towards higher values in Russian women.

The levels of autoantibodies to thyroid components were significantly higher in the population of Russian women, and the levels of autoantibodies to protein-lipid components of the haemostasis system, which characterise antiphospholipid reactions, were higher in the Tajik population, as was the blood clotting time in the lebetox test.

Since the main source of autoantibodies is the B_1 -subpopulation of lymphocytes [90], the blood content of this category of lymphocytes was monitored in women of both populations. . This study showed that the content of B_1 -lymphocytes in the blood of Tajik women is almost two times higher than in the Russian population, which pathogenetically can be associated with a higher predisposition of women of the Tajik population to autoimmune mune processes.

There were certain immunogenetic population differences, more pronounced in HLA class II gene loci. The genes associated with reproductive disorders in women - alleles HLA-DRB1*04, HLA-DQA1*103, HLA-DQA1*301, HLA-DQB1*302 - deserve special attention [11, 28]. Thus, the HLA-DRB1*04 allele was significantly more frequent in women of the Tajik population (1.4 times). The frequency of HLA-DQA1*0103 allele was significantly higher in Russian women (1.6-fold), and HLA-DQA1*0301 (1.5-fold) and HLA-DQB1*0302 (1.5-fold) alleles were significantly more frequent in Tajik women. These data suggest that the genetic nature of non-pregnancy is slightly more frequent in Tajik women.

The second objective of the study was to conduct cluster analysis in populations of Russian and Tajik women to identify features associated with favourable and unfavourable obstetric history based on informative immunogenetic, hormonal and immunological traits.

In the Russian population, 81 people were monitored, 28 of whom had all previous pregnancies ending in healthy births, and 53 of whom showed signs of reproductive health problems, as their obstetric history included either miscarriage, premature birth, foetal growth retardation or stillbirths. In the Tajik population, a similar study involved 85 women (28 with good reproductive health and 57 with reproductive disorders).

To conduct this section of the research, the most informative features that allow differentiating between women with preserved and impaired reproductive health were first established separately in both the Russian and Tajik populations using discrimi nant analysis. These characteristics were used in the cluster analysis programme to classify the data in each population.

Cluster 1 (aka group 1) in the population of Russian women consisted of reproductively healthy women, clusters 2 and 3 included women with pathological shifts in reproductive health, but differing in the sets of characteristic shifts in the indicators. In group 2, the most pronounced shifts were observed in immunological indicators: the number of lymphocytes with cytotoxic activity increased, and an increase in the content of IgG class antibodies to β2-glycoprotein was detected. In group 3 with reproductive pathology, hormonal shifts prevailed among the identified abnormalities: the blood content of estradiol, progesterone and prolactin was higher, while the level of autoantibodies to thyroglobulin was lower.

In the population of Tajik women there were also 3 clusters - groups 5, 6, 7. As in the case of Russian women, group 5 consisted of women with preserved reproductive function. Group 6 included women with reproductive dysfunction, who had a decrease in the level of informative sex hormones and one of their thyroid hormones, an increase in the level of cortisol, a selective increase in autoantibodies to thyroid proteins, as well as the main subpopulations of T-lymphocytes, network killers, B-lymphocytes, and IgG levels. Another part of women with reproductive disorders from cluster 7 was characterised by selective growth of IgG-antibodies to phospholipids, β_2 -glycoprotein and prothrombin.

In the process of solving this problem, immunogenetic studies were also conducted in clusters, which showed a higher occurrence of HLA-DQB1*0303 and HLA-DQB1*0503 alleles in Russian women with preserved reproductive function, while in the population of Tajik women HLA-DQB1*0302 and HLA-DQB1*0602-8 alleles were registered with a rather high and significantly different frequency.

Interestingly, according to our data, unfavourable alleles in both populations were associated with reproductive disorders regardless of the cluster affiliation of women. This rule was not absolute, because, for example, carriage of such alleles as DQA1*301 and DQB1*302 with a rather high frequency was also observed in women with preserved reproductive function, especially in the Tajik population.

These results require further more detailed analysis, as they suggest that not only HLA-DRB1*04, HLA-DQA1*0103, HLA-DQA1*301, HLA-DQB1*302 alleles may be genetic markers of reproductive disorders. The question of association with reproduction of such alleles as HLA-DRB1*01, HLA-DRB1*11, HLA-DRB1*13, HLA-DQA1*0501, HLA-DQB1*050, which can also claim to be markers of reproductive pathology, also needs special consideration. The question of the categories of those external and phenotypic conditions under which these genes may manifest their undesirable effects on reproductive function deserves separate consideration.

As for the cluster approach as a whole when combined with a population-based approach for determining the characteristics of reproductive health disorders, we have not encountered a similar method of grouping data in either domestic or foreign literature.

The next objective of the study was to characterise the hormonal status of women in the Russian and Tajik populations at risk of reproductive disorders in order to identify quantitative shifts in hormones associated with the reproductive process.

The data obtained showed that the nature of deviations in the content of sex hormones in the blood of women of the Russian and Tajik populations belonging to risk groups for reproductive dysfunction is ambiguous.

In the category of Russian women out of two risk groups, only one (group 3) shows a rather significant increase in the blood content of follicle mulating hormone, luteinising hormone, prolactin, estradiol, progesterone, thyroid hormone, total T3 and T4, which occurs against the background of a significant decrease in the levels of testosterone, its metabolite dihydroepiandro sterone, and cortisol. In the same group, a moderate decrease in the levels of autoantibodies to thyroid components was noted compared to healthy women In another risk group (group 2), the indicators of hormone content and antibodies to them almost completely correspond to those of healthy women.

In the category of Tajik women, reliable deviations from the control (indicators of healthy women) are of a different nature, although they also affect only one of the risk groups - Group 6. In this group, on the contrary, there is a significant drop in the blood content of all sex hormones except androgens (the level of the latter is increasing); their thyroid hormone levels are moderately reduced, but at the same time there is a rather significant increase in the blood content of autoantibodies to thyroid components; cortisol levels are elevated.

Despite the identified shifts, only a small group of hormones and antibodies to them can serve as markers of the risk group for the development of reproductive disorders in each population of women. This was established by determining 95% confidence intervals and constructing ROC curves of prognostic significance for each indicator of hormonal status in each of the 6 study groups.

As a result, a set of prognostically significant indicators of reproductive dysfunction and ranges of their values were determined, and the degree of their prognostic significance was established:

- for group 3 of the Russian population - luteinising hormone > 5.1 IU/l (AUROC = 0.935), prolactin > 136 mIU/ml (AUROC = 0.982), estradiol > 237 pmol/l (AUROC = 0.928), progesterone > 26.5 nmol/l (AUROC = 1.0), thyroid hormone > 1.6 mIU/l (AUROC = 0.982). 26.5 nmol/L (AUROC = 1.0), thyroid hormone > 1.6 mIU/L (AUROC = 0.982), total thyroxine > 86.5 nmol/L (AUROC = 1.0), cortisol < 291 nmol/L (AUROC = 0.982);

- for group 6 of Tajik population - prolactin < 140 nmol/l (AUROC = 0.933), estradiol < 240 pmol/l (AUROC = 0.880), progesterone < 30 nmol/l (AUROC = 0.915), autoantibodies to thyroglobulin > 80 ME/ml (AUROC = 0.985). 30 nmol/l (AUROC = 0.915), autoantibodies to thyroglobulin > 80 ME/ml (AUROC = 0.985), autoantibodies to thyroperoxidase > 40 ME/ml (AUROC = 1.0), cortisol > 330 nmol/l (AUROC = 0.933).

Another objective: to characterise the immune status of women in the Russian and Tajik populations at risk of reproductive disorders in order to identify quantitative shifts in immune system cells and immunoglobulins of different classes associated with the reproductive process.

This section of the study, as well as the previous one, consisted of two stages, the first was aimed at identifying risk groups for reproductive disorders involving immune mechanisms, and the second stage was aimed at determining prognostically significant risk criteria.

At the first stage, it was found that in the population of Russian women, the main immunophenotypic and immunoglobulin shifts were observed in group 2 with reproductive health disorders. while the main abnormalities in hormonal status were registered, as has already been noted, in group 3. As in group 3, immunological shifts of group 2 were registered within the reference range. The greatest upward deviations were observed in the cells potentially possessing cytotoxic activity - cytotoxic T-lymphocytes (CD3+CD8+), natural killer cells (CD16+CD56+), EKT (CD3+CD56+). A significant increase in the number of B-lymphocytes (CD19+) was also observed. Among the three classes of immunoglobulins, only IgG level showed sufficient (high) prognostic significance. In the same group the levels of total autoantibodies of IgG class to human phospholipids, IgG-autoantibodies to β_2 -glycoprotein, annexin V, prothrombin, blood content of lupus anticoagulant increased significantly.

In the population of Tajik women, reliable deviations were registered in group 6, and in the latter case, hormonal shifts were also registered in the same group. The main emphasis in the degree of deviation from the indicators of healthy women fell, first of all, on the lymphocytes of the innate immune response that take part in the realisation of reproductive function - natural killer cells (CD16+CD56+) and EKT (CD3+CD56+). The number of B-lymphocytes increased in parallel, which coincided in this category of examined women with the previously registered increase in the levels of autoantibodies to thyroid proteins. Significant deviations from the indicators of healthy women in group 6 were noted for all classes of immunoglobulins. In group 7, the levels of IgG class autoantibodies to human phospholipids, β_2 -glycoprotein-1, prothrombin, and blood clotting time in the lebetox test remained promising for further investigation as markers of reproductive health disorders.

Determination of the 95% confidence interval of the indicators and their prognostic significance in the form of ROC-curves allowed us to select informative markers among the marked deviations in both populations:

- in group 2 women of the Russian population - increase in the number of lymphocytes with phenotypes CD3+CD4+ > 35.7% (AUROC = 0.890), CD3+CD8+ > 20.2% (AUROC = 1.0), CD3+CD56+ > 4.2% (AUROC = 0.967), CD16+CD56+ > 14.6% (AUROC = 1.0), CD19+ > 9.3% (AUROC = 0.968), increased IgG levels > 10.6 mg/ml (AUROC = 0.927);

- in group of 6 women of Tajik population - increase in the number of lymphocytes with phenotypes CD3+CD4+ > 33.2% (AUROC = 0.942), CD3+CD56+ > 2.2% (AUROC = 0.915), CD16+CD56+ > 13.8% (AUROC = 1.0), CD19+ > 14.2% (AUROC = 0.964), as well as an increase in IgG > 12.8 mg/ml (AUROC = 0.954) and a fall in CD3+CD8+ lymphocyte count < 19.2% (AUROC = 0.804).

The fifth objective of the study was to characterise the autoimmune compo nent in women of the Russian and Tajik populations at risk of reproductive disorders in order to identify quantitative shifts in autoantibodies potentially affecting the reproductive process.

Antiphospholipid reactions as an autoimmune state of hypercoagulability caused by antiphospholipid antibodies are closely associated with pregnancy pathology in a certain proportion of women with impaired reproductive health - [36, 114, 205].

In Russian women, an increase in the values of antiphospholipid reaction indicators was noted in group 2 with reproductive health disorders. In this group, the levels of total autoantibodies of IgG class to human phospholipids, IgG-autoantibodies to β_2 -glycoprotein, annexin V, prothrombin, and blood content of lupus anticoagulant increased significantly.

In Tajik women, the list of deviations of antiphospholipid reactions from healthy women extended to all autoimmune parameters, except for IgG-autoantibodies to annexin V and lupus anticoagulant determined in the lupus test.

Determination of the 95% confidence interval of the indicators and their prognostic significance in the form of ROC-curves allowed us to select informative markers among the marked deviations in both populations:

- in group 2 women of the Russian population - an increase in blood levels of autoantibodies to phospholipids > 3.6 U/ml (AUROC = 0.971) and β_2 -glycoprotein1 > 4.8 U/ml (AUROC = 1.0);

- in group of 7 women of Tajik population - increase in the blood content of total IgG-autoantibodies to phospholipids > 9 U/ml (AUROC = 0.993). 9 U/ml (AUROC = 0.993), IgG-autoantibodies to β_2 - glycoprotein I > 8 U/ml (AUROC = 1.0), IgG-autoantibodies to prothrombin > 8.7 U/ml (AUROC = 0.988).

Finally, the last task of the study was to create a system of integral risk assessment of reproductive health disorders in women of the Russian and Tajik populations, to develop algorithms for its use, and to test this system on a cohort of unborn women with subsequent follow-up in catamnesis.

First of all, it was shown that the use of risk criteria for reproductive disorders obtained in previous studies is not always effective. For example, a total of 8 markers were selected for group 2 of the population of Russian women with predominant immunological shifts. At the same time, all these markers were noted in 22 people (82%) of group 2, 1 person of this group (4%) had 6 markers out of 8 and 4 people of group 2 had 5 markers out of 8.

Markers of risk group 6 in the population of Tajik women are significantly higher in frequency of occurrence in this group and in no case show a value below 70%. In all other groups, the frequency of occurrence of these markers, as a rule, is in the range of 1-8%, although in some cases reaching 24-47%.

The few markers in risk group 7 are even more effective in recognising whether women belong to this group. In group 7 itself, the frequency of occurrence of these markers is between 93% and 100%, while in the other groups it does not exceed 4%.

In addition, we proceeded from the assumption that the influence of each criterion indicator on reproductive health is unequal and it is reasonable to use the principle of integral assessment to predict women's risk of reproductive disorders.

For this purpose, a regression analysis was performed for each risk group, in which all laboratory parameters capable of exhibiting marker properties for reproductive disorders were included.

For risk group 2, a linear regression equation of the following kind was obtained: 0.257*[number of CTLs] + 0.266*[number of ECs] + + 0.122*[number of B-lf] + 0.107*[level of IgG] + 0.209*[level of AT to β_2 -GP]. In the process of obtaining the regression equation, the statistical programme excluded 3 indicators (the number of T-helpers, the number of ECT and the level of antibodies to human phospholipids), and of the remaining 5 blood indicators, the number of cytotoxic T-lymphocytes, the number of natural killer cells and the level of IgG-autoantibodies to β_2 -glycoproteins were the most informative, judging by the value of weight coefficients. As a result, in each case an index was obtained, which we hereinafter denoted as the integral marker of reproductive impairment 1 (IMNR1).

Then, in women of all studied groups, the data corresponding to 5 informative markers of group 2 were substituted into the regression equation. As a result, individual values of the integral marker of reproductive disorders 1 were obtained in each case.

By determining the 95% confidence interval and constructing the ROC-curve, the following was established. Determination of the integral marker on the basis of a linear regression equation makes it possible to bring the predictive value of the test almost to the absolute value (AUROC = 1.0). A more detailed analysis using the standard deviations of the 95% confidence interval showed that the maximum of deviations in the comparison groups was 11.5 and, therefore, the value of IMNR1 above 11.5 was prognostically significant in terms of the possibility of reproductive disorders.

Similarly, integral markers of reproductive disorders were calculated for all other risk groups.

For risk group 3 of the population of Russian women, a regression equation of the following form was obtained: 0.341*[prolactin] + 0.257*[estradiol] + + 0.184*[total T4] - 0.153*[cortisol]. In this case, three indicators were excluded from the formula by the statistical programme - levels of luteinising hormone, progesterone, thyroid hormone, and the remaining 4 indicators were included in the regression equation, with prolactin (coefficient 0.341) and estradiol (coefficient 0.257) being the most informative.

The calculation of IMNR2 by solving this linear regression equation yielded a diagnostic test whose predictive value was extremely high (AUROC = 0.996) at values above 85, i.e. at these values of IMNR2, a woman can reasonably be classified as a risk group for reproductive health disorders associated with hormonal shifts.

In the risk group 5 population of Tajik women associated with hormonal-immunological signs of reproductive health disorders, regression analysis yielded a regression equation that included only 2 immunological indicators out of 12: -9.049 + 0.537*[EC count] - 0.208*[B-lymphocyte count].

Calculation and subsequent analysis of the IMNR3 derived from this regression equation showed that, with a value above 14, the predictive value of such a test was close to absolute, as AUROC = 1.0.

Regression analysis was also performed for risk group 6 based on the characteristic for this group increase in the values of IgG-autoantibodies to human phospholipids (HPA), β_2 -glycoproteins, prothrombin. The regression equation obtained was as follows: 2.179 + 0.288*[AFA] + 0.453*[AT to β_2 -GP].

This regression equation included only two out of three indicators, because the level of IgG-autoantibodies to prothrombin was not involved in the formation of the intergal marker of reproductive disorders (IMNR4). The individual values of each woman who participated in the study were then substituted into the regression equation. The integral marker of reproductive disorders in group 6 (IMNR4), as in all other cases, distinguished with almost absolute clarity (AUROC = 1.0) the belonging of women to this group with a value higher than 8.5.

In order to make sure once again how effectively the integral indicators of IMNR1-IMNR2 for Russian women and IMNR3-IMNR4 for Tajik women developed in this section of the research can be applied in medical practice, they were tested in groups of unborn women of each population.

A long-term (three-year) follow-up of 30 unmarried women in the Russian population planning pregnancy (group 4) showed the following. Four women who did not become pregnant during the next three years were subsequently excluded from the study, as this phenomenon may be based on disorders of not only female but also male reproductive health or a high degree of concordance between the genotypes of the couple. All tested parameters of the remaining 26 women in Group 4 were fully within the reference ranges, and both regression equations were calculated for them in order to determine integral markers of reproductive health disorders 1 and 2 (IMNR1 and IMNR2).

Twenty-one pregnancies resulted in the birth of a healthy child, and in two cases even two children. Four women experienced pregnancy failure (in one case it was combined with a second pregnancy that ended safely), and one woman had premature labour with loss of a child. Determination of the integral marker of reproductive disorders associated with predominant shifts in immune status (IMNR1) allowed us to assign a woman to the risk group in only one case (IMNR1>11.5). This woman developed preterm labour at 28 weeks and the foetus could not be saved. Four women with miscarriage had high BMI2 values (>85) associated with hormonal shifts. In other words, in these cases, IMNR2 values clearly indicated the possibility of hormone-mediated reproductive dysfunction, although the hormonal status indicators in this case were within the reference values.

In a similar study in the Tajik population, the integral measures of IMNR3 and IMNR4 were tested on a specially selected group of 32 unmarried Tajik women (group 8) who, as in the Russian population, were followed up by an obstetrician-gynaecologist for the next 3 years. This cohort was composed of young women planning pregnancy. However, 3 women did not become pregnant during the first year of follow-up and were referred for further evaluation and excluded from the cohort, while the remaining women were followed up.

Twenty-five women in the Tajik population, who had not had a pregnancy before the study, developed pregnancies (and in 6 cases even 2) within the next 3 years and gave birth to healthy children. At the same time, none of the women with preserved reproductive function had values of IMNR3 > 14.0 and/or IMNR4 > 8.5, which are characteristic of reproductive disorders.

Four women in the Tajik population had reproductive health disorders. In three cases, it was manifested by pregnancy failure, which coincided with relatively high values of IMNR3 (14.4 and 14.7) and IMNR4 (8.7), and in one case the pregnancy ended in preterm labour with IMNR4 = 8.8.

Based on these findings, we proposed algorithms for screening women in both populations.

According to these algorithms, it is recommended that women in the Russian population be examined on days 3-5 of the menstrual cycle, as the examination scheme includes such hormones as oestradiol and prolactin, which are determined at these times. Women in the Tajik population can be examined regardless of the timing of the menstrual cycle.

The venous blood of women is analysed by solid-phase immunoenzyme analysis and flow cytofluorimetry for the indicators included in the formulas for calculating IMNR1/IMNR2 in the Russian population and IMNR3/IMNR4 in the Tajik population.

Next, integral indicators are calculated and evaluated according to the recommended ranges of values. If at least one of the indicators falls within the prognostically significant range of values, the woman is placed in the risk group for possible reproductive health disorders.

Thus, the research conducted creates a reliable basis for the possibility of predicting health disorders in the populations of both Russian and Tajik women at the prenosological stage. This became possible due to the development of an original methodological approach to grouping data on the basis of population cluster analysis.

Moreover, the obtained data, although characterising the study as a completed scientific work, open the prospect for a number of new directions of research. One of them concerns the correspondence of immunogenetic features of reproductive disorders to the other shifts. Another possible direction concerns analysing which reproductive disorders correspond to each variant in their risk assessment. In the future, it will also be necessary to establish what mechanisms underlie the reported reproductive variants, provided that the observed shifts are within the physiological normal range.

CONCLUSIONS

1. Average regional norms of hormonal status in clinically healthy women of reproductive age living in Tajikistan and the Central Chernozem region of Russia have been established and scientifically substantiated.It is shown that within the physiological fluctuations of hormonal status, the average level of gonadotropic hormones FSH, LH, P, E, PL in Tajik women was lower than in Russian women, respectively, by 20.0, 18.0, 36.0, 16.6, and 32.2%; the level of thyroid hormones TTG, total T3, and total T4 was also lower in Tajik women, respectively, by 48.2, 24.0, and 20.0%. It was found that the average regional norms of androgens and glucocorticosteroids in Tajik women were higher than in Russian women: cortisol by 16.0 per cent, testosterone by 21.0 per cent, 17-OP by 30.0 per cent, DHEA-C by 25.5 per cent.

2. Average regional norms of cellular and humoral immunity indices have been established and scientifically substantiated. It is shown that in Russian women the average regional indicators of cellular immunity were higher than similar indicators in Tajik women: cytotoxic T-suppressor cells (CD3/8+) by 31.7%; cells with killer activity NK-cells (CD56) by 26.6%; NK-cells (CD16) by 43.4%; NK-cells (CD3/16/56+) by 57.1%; NK-cells (CD3-/16/56+) by 16.6%; NK-cells (CD3/56/16-) by 8.0%. At the same time, in Tajik girls, the average regional indicators of B-lymphocytes (CD19+) were higher by 51.6%, B-cells (CD19/CD5+) by 46.1%. At the same time, immunoglobulin IgA was lower by 40.0%, IgG higher by 18.0%.

3. It was found that the average regional indicators of markers of AFR in Tajik women were significantly higher than those of Russian women. Thus, APA was higher by 58.2%, β-2-glycoprotein by 50.0%, Annexin-V by 56.8%, Prothrombin by 44.6%, APTV by 20.0% and Clotting Time by 44.0%. It is shown that compared to the average regional norm, an increased level of AT-antibodies to thyroid hormones was found in 30.5% of Russian women. Carriage of AT-TPO was detected in 21.9 per cent of the women examined, and AT-TG in 8.1 per cent. In Tajik women, elevated levels of AT-antibodies were detected in 10.5 per cent, AT-TPO in 6.9 per cent and AT-TG in 3.1 per cent of women.

4. The population cluster approach, based on the use of discri mi nant and cluster analysis, is a highly effective way of grouping women according to their reproductive health status and the risk factors that caused reproductive disorders

5. The risk factors causing reproductive disorders are different in combination in the populations of Russian and Tajik women, including a greater frequency of allelic variants of HLA-DRB1*04, HLA-DQA1*0301, HLA-DQB1*0302 in the Tajik population and HLA-DQA1*0103 in the Russian population.

6. In the population of Russian women with reproductive disorders, two risk groups are distinguished at the prenosological stage, one of which is characterised by changes in the hormonal status of luteinising hormone, prolactin, oestradiol, progesterone, thyroo tropic hormone, total thyroxine, cortisol, and the other -

immunological shifts, including the number of lymphocytes with phenotypes CD3+CD4+, CD3+CD8+, CD3+CD56+, CD16+CD56+, CD19+, IgG level, blood content of autoantibodies to phospholipids and β_2 -glycoprotein-1 in quantitative ranges typical for this population.

7. In the population of Tajik women with reproductive disorders, there are 2 risk groups, one of which is characterised by changes in the hormonal-immune status of prolactin, oestradiol, progesterone, cortisol, levels of autoantibodies to thyrogl bulin, thyroperoxidase, number of lymphocytes with phenotypes CD3+CD4+, CD3+CD8+, CD3+CD56+, CD16+CD56+, CD19+, IgG level, and the other - autoimmune shifts including levels of IgG-autoantibodies to phospho lipids, β_2 -glycoprotein, prothrombin in quantitative ranges typical for this population.

8. In a population of Russian women, reproductive disorders associated with immunological shifts can be identified and predicted by the value of the integral marker IMNR1 > 11.5, calculated by the formula: 0.257*[number of CTLs] + 0.266*[number of ECs] + 0.122*[number of B-lymphocytes] + 0.107*[level of IgG] + 0.209*[level of autoantibodies to β_2 -glycoprotein].

9. In the population of Russian women, reproductive disorders associated with hormonal shifts can be identified and predicted by the value of the integral marker IMNR2 > 85, calculated by the formula: 0.341*[prolactin] + 0.257*[estradiol] + 0.014*[TSH] + + + 0.184*[total T4] - 0.153*[cortisol].

10. In a population of Tajik women, reproductive disorders associated with hormonal and immunological shifts can be identified and predicted by the value of the integral marker IMNR3 > 14, calculated by the formula: -9.049 + 0.537*[number of EC] - 0.208*[number of B-lymphocytes].
11. In a population of Tajik women, reproductive disorders associated with the development of antiphospholipid reactions can be identified and predicted by the value of the integral marker IMNR4 > 8.5, calculated by the formula: 2.179 + 0.288*[level of autoantibodies to phospholipids] + 0.453*[level of autoantibodies to β_2 -glycoprotein].

PRACTICAL RECOMMENDATIONS

1. When introducing new laboratory technologies related to the identification fica of signs of reproductive health disorders in women of fertile age at the prenosological stage, it is advisable to use a cluster-population methodological approach.
2. In the study of physiological functions of certain ethnic groups and populations of women, it is necessary to clarify the reference ranges of laboratory values.
3. Given the multifactorial nature of the causes of reproductive disorders in women of fertile age, when developing an algorithm for predicting these disorders, preference should be given to integral markers of reproductive disorders, developed, for example, using regression data analysis.
4. In order to predict reproductive health disorders in women of fertile age in the Russian population, it is advisable to use our proposed integral indicators IMNR1 and IMNR2, with IMNR1 contributing to the detection of the risk of reproductive disorders of immune genesis, and IMNR2 - the risk of reproductive disorders of hormonal genesis.
5. To predict reproductive health disorders in women of fertile age in the Tajik population, it is advisable to use our proposed integral indicators IMNR3 and IMNR4, with IMNR3 helping to identify the risk of reproductive disorders of hormonal and immune genesis, and IMNR2 - the risk of reproductive disorders due to the threat of antiphospholipid reactions.
6. To predict reproductive health disorders in women of fertile age in the Russian and Tajik populations, it is advisable to use the relevant algorithms developed in this study.

REFERENCE LIST

1. Aghajanyan N.A., Manapova I.I. Ethnic aspect of adaptation physiology and morbidity of the population // Human Ecology. - 2014. - № 3. - C. 3-13.

2. Azimova M.K.. Impact of atmospheric air pollution on women's reproductive health //Biology and Integrative Medicine 2016, 1(1), 64-69.

3. Aleksandrova EM, Botasheva TL, Ermolova NV, Khloponina AV, Pligina EV Influence of ethnic characteristics on the adaptation processes of the female body in the reproductive period // Medical Bulletin of the South of Russia, 2013. - № 4. - C. 5-8.

4. Anoshkina N.L., Gulin A.V. Some aspects of health and physical development of students of a large industrial centre // Medico-social problems of modern Russia. Moscow, 2008, P.10-14.

5. Apolikhin O.I., Moskaleva N.G., Komarova V.A. Modern demographic situation and problems of improving reproductive health of the Russian population // Experimental and Clinical Urology, 2015. - № 4. - C. 4-14.

6. Arabzoda S.N., Shukurov F.A. Activity of the stress-realising system in students in the process of their education // Bulletin of the Academy of Medical Sciences of Tajikistan. 2016. № 4. C. 19-23.

7. Arabzoda S.N., Shukurov F.A., Melikova N.H. Psychovegetative status in the assessment of adaptive capacity to emotional stress // Applied Information Aspects of Medicine. 2015. T. 18. № 1. C. 32-37.

8. Arabova Z.U., Nevzorova E.V. pH of arterial blood in humans under conditions of high-altitude hypoxaemia // Bulletin of the Polessky State University. - 2013. - PART 1. - P. 7-9

9. Arabova Z.U., Nevzorova EV, Shukurov FA, Gulin AV Change in electrolyte concentrations in hypoxia // Vestnik of Tambov University. Series: Natural and Technical Sciences. 2013. T. 18. № 6-2. C. 3283-3285.

10. Arabova Z.U., Shukurov F.A. Prediction of the optimal duration of human habitation at high altitudes In the collection: Ecological and physiological problems of adaptation. Materials of

XVIII All-Russian symposium with international participation. Peoples' Friendship University of Russia. 2019. C. 28-30.

11. Arabova Z.U., Shukurov F.A. State of the autonomous nervous system in the assessment of human adaptation to high-mountain hypoxia // Applied Information Aspects of Medicine. 2015. T. 18. № 1. C. 73-75.

12. Arabova Z.U., Shukurov F.A., Malysheva E.V. Evaluation of oxygenation parameters in high altitude conditions // Bulletin of Tambov University. Series: Natural and Technical Sciences. - 2012. - Vol. 17, Vyp. 4. - C. 1282-1285.

13. Arabova Z.U., Shukurov F.A., Nevzorova E.V. Parameters of acid-base state of blood in the assessment of high-altitude hypoxaemia // Bulletin of Lipetsk State Pedagogical University. - 2013 - MIFE Series, Vol. 1 (4). - C. 58-66.

14. Akhmedov A.A., Bobokhodjaeva M.O., Nazirova M.A. et al. Trends in fertility in the Republic of Tajikistan in the new economic conditions // Health Care of Tajikistan, 2010. - № 2 - C. 5-11

15. Akhmedov K.Y., Shukurov F.A. Relationship of heart rate parameters with physical performance of people during adaptation to high-mountain hypoxia // Human Physiology. 1984. T. 8. № 6. C. 943.

16. Akhmedov F.K. Study of the role of renal blood flow and uric acid concentration in blood and urine in the diagnosis of pre-eclampsia// Theoretical and Clinical Medicine. - 2015. - №3. - C. 63-66.

17. Akhmedov F.K., Negmatullaeva M.N. Uric acid as a pathogenic factor in pre-eclampsia //Biology and Integrative Medicine 2020, 6(46), 31-40.

18. Ashurova N.G., Bobokulova S.B. Study of menstrual function in adolescent schoolgirls //Biology and Integrative Medicine 2021, 6(53), 30-35.

19. Ashurova N.G., Mavlonova G.Sh. Role of hormonal status of reproductive system recovery at pubertal age // New Day of Medicine. - 2018. - №3. - C. 57-59.

20. Babadjanova G.S., Tukhtamisheva N.O. Modern view on the diagnosis and treatment of uterine myoma in women of reproductive age //Biology and Integrative Medicine 2017, 2(8), 64-79.

21. Badritdinova MN, Kudratova D.Sh., Ochilova D.A. Prevalence of some components of metabolic syndrome in the

female population //Biology and Integrative Medicine 2016, 2(2), 53-61.

22. Badritdinova MN, Tukhtaev DA Frequency of occurrence of risk factors of carbohydrate metabolism disorders in patients with hypertension //Biology and Integrative Medicine 2021, 5(52), 58-64.

23. Baevsky R.M. Physiological norm and the concept of health //Russian Physiological Journal. 2003, T.89, 4, 473-489.

24. Balmukhamedova J.A., Zemlyanskaya N.S., Derbisalina G.A. Subclinical left ventricular dysfunction in women in the menopausal period //Biology and Integrative Medicine 2021, 6(53), 36-43.

25. Boldonosova NA, Druzhinina EB. Folliculo- and oogenesis: chemical properties and biological action of luteinising hormone // Siberian Medical Journal, 2014. - T. 129, № 6. - C. 28-31.

26. Borisova O.I. Comparative ecological-physiological characteristic of dependence of reproductive function of women on the level of anthropotechnogenic load // Avicenna Bulletin, 2008, 2 (35), 22-25.

27. Gadzhieva IA, Chistyakova GN Violation of immune regulation at the stage of placentation as a cause of reproductive losses // Problems of Reproduction, 2011, 4, 102-107

28. Gulzoda K., Halimova F.T., Shukurov F.A. Ethnicity and reproductive health - a cluster-population approach to assessing the reproductive health of women of fertile age LAP LAMBERT, Mauritius, 2019, 305

29. Gulin A.V., Shukurov F.A., Halimova F.T. Reproductive health of women of different ethnic groups //Biology and Integrative Medicine 2019, 9(37), 4-67.

30. Danishevsky K.D. Reproductive health: global development goals and economic potential of Russia //Medicine, 2013. - N 2. - C. 13-28.

31. Dobrohotova Yu.E., Dzhobava E.M., Ozerova R.I. Non-developing pregnancy: thromboembolic and clinical and immunological factors M.: GEOTAR-Media, 2010, 144 pp.

32. Elifanov A.V. Lepunova O.N. The level of gonadotropic and sex hormones in some forms of endocrine infertility in women // Bulletin of Tyumen State University, 2014, No. 6, 114-122.

33. Ermenteva L.N., Aitbaeva J.B., Akpolatova G.M. The effect of "mediator substances" fetal cell on changes in the activity

of serum transaminase enzymes in rats after lethal hypobaric hypoxia //Biology and Integrative Medicine 2016, 4(4), 5-14.

34. Zakhryapina L.V. Regional peculiarities of endocrine disorders in women of fertile age in conditions of different levels of anthropotechnogenic load of the territory of resident residence // Uspekhi sovremennomennoi naukhestvosnaniya, 2010, 3, 37-39.

35. Kalachikova O.N. Trends and prospects of reproductive behaviour of the population (on the example of the Vologda Oblast). Cand. ekon. nauk. Moscow, 2013. - 24 c.

36. Karomatov I.D., Takaeva Sh.K. Application of bee royal jelly in diseases of the urogenital system in men and women // Biology and Integrative Medicine 2020, 3(43), 137-154.

37. Kiseleva AN, Zaitseva GA, Isaeva NV, Butina EV Features of polymorphism of genes of the HLA system in disorders of reproduction // **International** Research Journal, 2015, 7-5(38), 23-24.

38. Kozlov A.I. Changes in the gene pool of northern populations: "sunset of ethnoses" or formation of a new adaptive group? // Bulletin of Archaeology, Anthropology and Ethnography, 2014, Vol. 3, 26, 99-107.

39. Komilzhanova D.K. The role of antiphospholipid syndrome in the prevention of pregnancy failure //Biology and Integrative Medicine 2017, 5(11), 21-27.

40. Konovalova S.G., Conteeva N.A. Ecological morphology of the feto-placental system (literature review) // Human Ecology, 2005, 2, 17-24.

41. Labygina AV, Zagarskikh EY, Darjaev ZY, Shipkhineeva TI Thyroid disease and reproductive health of the female population of the main ethnic groups of Eastern Siberia // Bulletin of the East Siberian Scientific Centre SB RAS, 2013, 92, 41-45.

42. Laptina T.A. Immunogenetics and human reproduction Rostov-on-Don, 2013. 80 c.

43. Leonova Z.A., Florensov V.V.. Synthesis and functions of female sex hormones // Siberian Medical Journal, 2013, 2, 10-13.

44. Marinkin I.O., Kuleshov V.M., Galkina Y.V., Aidagulova S.V. Correction of neuroobmeno-endocrine syndrome in women of reproductive age // Medicine and Education in Siberia, 2012, 2, 65-66.

45. Mindubaeva F.A., Shukurov F.A., Salikhova E.Y. Ethnic features of adaptive reactions of students living in different climatic and geographical conditions / In the collection: Heart rhythm and type of vegetative regulation in assessing the level of public health and functional fitness of athletes. Proceedings of the VI All-Russian symposium. 2016. C. 209-213.

46. Mukhamadieva S.M., Nirzabekova B.T., Usmanova F.I. Clinical manifestations of climacteric syndrome in meno- and postmenopausal women// Reports of the Academy of Sciences of the Republic of Tajikistan, 2007. T. 50, 1, 79-84.

47. Nabieva F.C. Modern aspects of epidemiology, etiology and diagnosis of ovarian cancer (literature review) //Biology and Integrative Medicine 2016, 2(2), 110-131.

48. Nikolaeva V.V., Shukurov F.A. Ethnic characteristics of growth and weight of girls in the Hissar Valley of Tajikistan //Biology and Integrative Medicine 2020, 6(46), 23-30.

49. Orziev Z.M., Suleymanova G.T. Regional causes of iron deficiency anaemia in women of fertile age //Biology and Integrative Medicine 2018, 4(21), 74-82.

50. Pakhomov S.P. Regional peculiarities of women's reproductive health and the factors contributing to their formation. Doctor of medical sciences. Moscow, 2006. - 41 c.

51. Pisareva E.V., Razumnaya A.E., Borzenkova A.V. Studies of the hormonal status of women with various reproductive disorders // Bulletin of SamSMU - Natural Science Series, 2013, 9/1 (110), 197.

52. Rakhimova Z.A. Optimisation of diagnostic methods for various forms of adenomyosis in women of reproductive age //Biology and Integrative Medicine 2016, 5(5), 48-53.

53. Rakhmatova D., Karomatov I.D. Phytotherapy in the prevention and treatment of premenstrual syndrome //Biology and Integrative Medicine 2018, 11(28), 93-104.

54. Rakhmatullaeva M.M. Microecological aspects of women's reproductive health// Almanac of Young Science. Orenburg. - 2018, №4, 24-30.

55. Russkova AN, Kosynkina T.M. Antiphospholipid syndrome - one of the variants of violation of the relationship between the regulatory systems // International Journal of Applied and Basic Research, 2012, 1, 69.

56. Tananakina TP, Lysenko EA, Zadorozhny SP, Parinov RA, Kutsevol OV Comparative index assessment of the

physical state of the organism of young men and girls students of medical universities studying in different socio-economic conditions //Biology and Integrative Medicine 2021, 6(53), 350-358.

57. Tuksanova D.I. Structural and geometric changes in left ventricular function in pregnant women with pre-eclampsia //Biology and Integrative Medicine 2020, 6(46), 49-58.

58. Tuksanova D.I., Negmatullaeva MN Doppler echocardiography in the course of pre-eclampsia on the background of chronic hypertension //Biology and Integrative Medicine 2020, 3(43), 24-35.

59. Khalimova F.T. Hormonal profile in women of reproductive age of different ethnic groups / Health of the population - the basis of prosperity of Russia, Materials of the X Anniversary All-Russian scientific-practical conference with international participation. Branch of RGSU in Anapa. 2016, 322-324

60. Halimova F.T. Thyroid and adrenal hormones in predicting the risk group of violation of women's reproductive health / Proceedings of the XXIII Congress of the I.P. Pavlov Physiological Society with international participation, Moscow, 2017, 201-202

61. Halimova F.T. Immuno-genetic markers of hereditary predisposition to antiphospholipid reaction // Bulletin of the Academy of Medical Sciences of Tajikistan 2017, 4(24), 78-81

62. Halimova F.T. Cluster approach to the assessment of women's reproductive health //Vestnik of the Academy of Medical Sciences of Tajikistan 2017, 2(22), 72-76

63. Halimova F.T. Hereditary predisposition to antiphospholipid reaction /Ecological and physiological problems of adaptation - materials of XVIII All-Russian symposium with international participation. Peoples' Friendship University of Russia. 2019, 239-241

64. Halimova F.T. Features of gonadotropic and thyroid hormones in women living in different climatogeographical zones / Agajanianov Readings - materials of the II All-Russian scientific-practical conference with international participation. Peoples' Friendship University of Russia. Moscow, 2018, 271-272

65. Halimova F.T. Features of indicators of antiphospholipid reaction in women living in different climatogeographical zones //Vestnik of the Academy of Medical Sciences of Tajikistan 2018, 8, 1(25), 98-103

66. Halimova F.T. Features of the average regional indicators of cellular immunity in women living in different climatogeographical conditions // Vestnik of Tambov University. Series: Natural and Technical Sciences 2017, 22, 1, 217-220

67. Halimova F.T. Evaluation of thyroid system in women of different ethnic groups taking into account climatogeographical conditions of residence //Health, Demography, Ecology of Finno-Ugric Peoples 2015, 4, 88-91

68. Halimova F.T. Indicators of immunogenetic profile in the assessment of reproductive health of women living in different climatic and geographical zones // Bulletin of the Academy of Medical Sciences of Tajikistan 2016, 3, 114-119

69. Halimova F.T. Population features in women of fertile age /Ecological and physiological problems of adaptation - materials of the XVII All-Russian symposium with international participation. Peoples' Friendship University of Russia. 2017, 274-275

70. Halimova F.T. Epigenetic factors in the diagnosis of reproductive disorders // Bulletin of the Academy of Medical Sciences of Tajikistan 2017, 3(23), 91-97

71. Khalimova F.T., Abdusattorova M.A. State of reproductive health according to the indicators of cellular autoimmunity /Agadzhanyanov Readings - materials of the II All-Russian scientific-practical conference with international participation. Peoples' Friendship University of Russia. Moscow, 2018, 273-274.

72. Khalimova F.T., Ganizoda M.H., Abdusattorova M.A. Immunophysiological features of reproductive health development of antiphospholipid syndrome /Ecological and physiological problems of adaptation - materials of XVIII All-Russian symposium with international participation. Peoples' Friendship University of Russia. 2019, 241-243.

73. Halimova F.T., Gulin A.V., Malysheva E.V., Nazirova A.A. Clinical and laboratory characteristics of antiphospholipid syndrome in women with an obstetric history // Vestnik of Tambov University. Series: Natural and Technical Sciences 2012, 17, 4, 1285-1288.

74. Halimova F.T., Gulin A.V., Malysheva E.V., Nazirova A.A. Characteristics of blood coagulation parameters in antiphospholipid syndrome // Vestnik of Tambov University. Series: Natural and Technical Sciences 2102, 17, 5, 1449-1451

75. Halimova F.T., Gulin A.V., Nevzorova E.V., Nazirova A.A., Shukurov F.A. Determination of the criterion values of reproductive hormones in the formation of the risk group of reproductive disorders // Bulletin of Tambov University. Series: Natural and Technical Sciences. 2015. T. 20. № 6. C. 1640-1643.

76. Halimova F.T., Gulin A.V., Nevzorova E.V., Nazirova A.A., Shukurov F.A. Evaluation of reproductive hormonal profile in women of different ethnic groups, taking into account climatic and geographical conditions of residence // Vestnik of Tambov University. Series: Natural and Technical Sciences. 2015. T. 20. № 6. C. 1644-1648.

77. Halimova F.T., Gulin A.V., Nevzorova E.V., Shukurov F.A. Ethnic peculiarities of the immunogenetic profile of women living in different climatogeographical zones // In Proceedings: Health of the population - the basis of prosperity of Russia. Materials of X Jubilee All-Russian scientific-practical conference with international participation. Branch of RGSU in Anapa. 2016. C. 325-328.

78. Halimova F.T., Gulin A.V., Shukurov F.A. Features of the average regional indicators of hormonal profile in women living in different climatogeographical conditions // Vestnik of Tambov University. Series: Natural and Technical Sciences. 2016. T. 21. № 6. C. 2289-2294.

79. Halimova F.T., Gulin A.V., Shukurov F.A. Characteristics of humoral autoimmunity in women of different ethnic groups // Health, Demography, Ecology of Finno-Ugric Peoples 2015, 4, 91-93

80. Halimova F.T., Nevzorova E.V., Gulin A.V., Nazirova A.A. Immunoreactivity of the body of women of reproductive age living in the Lipetsk region // In the World of Scientific Discoveries. 2014. № 2 (50). C. 353-359

81. Halimova F.T., Nevzorova E.V., Gulin A.V., Nazirova A.A. Determination of the regional norm of immunological parameters in women of fertile age living in the Lipetsk region // Vestnik of Tambov University. Series: Natural and Technical Sciences 2013, 18, 6-2, 3286-3288.

82. Halimova F.T., Nevzorova E.V., Gulin A.V., Nazirova A.A., Shutova S.V. Characteristics of the immune status of women living in the Republic of Tajikistan / Actual problems of natural sciences -

materials of the International extramural scientific-practical conference. otv. 2014, 118-123.

83. Halimova F.T., Nevzorova E.V., Gulin A.V., Shukurov F.A. Comparative characteristics of the immunogenetic profile of women in Tajikistan and the Central Black Earth region of Russia // Vestnik of Tambov University. Series: Natural and Technical Sciences. 2016. T. 21. № 1. C. 231-235.

84. Halimova F.T., Nevzorova E.V., Gulin A.V., Shutova S.V. Determination of lupus-type anticoagulants in the assessment of antiphospholipid syndrome /Actual Problems of Natural Sciences 2013, 19-24.

85. Halimova FT, Nevzorova EV, Shukurov FA, Gulin AV Determination of the predictive value of IGG to prothrombin in relation to the assessment of antiphospholipid syndrome // In Proceedings: Health for All. Collection of articles of the V International Scientific and Practical Conference. Editorial Board: K.K. Shebcko [et al]. 2013. C. 267-268.

86. Halimova FT, Nevzorova EV, Shukurov FA, Gulin AV Role of proteins - cofactors in the development of antiphospholipid syndrome // Herald of Lipetsk State Pedagogical University. Series MIFE: Mathematics, Information Technologies, Physics, Natural Science 2013, 1(4), 113-115.

87. Halimova FT, Nevzorova EV, Shukurov FA, Gulin AV Comparative characteristics of reproductive immunophenotype and serum immunoglobulin levels in women of different ethnic groups // Vestnik of Lipetsk State Pedagogical University. Series MIFE: Mathematics, Information Technologies, Physics, Natural Science 2015, 1(16), 115-119.

88. Halimova F.T., Shukurov F.A. Hormonal status in the assessment of reproductive health disorders //Biology and Integrative Medicine 2019, 10(38), 4-12.

89. Halimova F.T., Shukurov F.A., Arabzoda S.N. Comparative characteristics of different forms of aggression with anxiety, correlation rhythmograms and functional state of the body //Vestnik of the Academy of Medical Sciences of Tajikistan 2020, 10, 2(34), 196-201.

90. Khalimova F.T., Shukurov F.A., Gulin A.V. Immuno-endocrine aspects of reproductive health of women of different ethnic groups (literature review) // In the book: HUMAN SCIENCE - FROM AVICENNA TO MODERNITY. Aslonova I.J., Aslonova Sh.J., Baimuradov R.R., Vorobeychik Y.N., Gulin

A.V., Karomatov I.D., Mavlonov A.A., Orziev Z.M., Orzieva Sh.Z., Ochilova D.A., Porsoev J.A., Ruziev O.A., Saidov S.A., Khaidarov N.K., Khaidarova D.K., Halimova F.T., Hodjaeva D.T., Sharipova D.S., Shukurov F.A. Bukhara, 2018. C. 4-69.

91. Halimova F.T., Shukurov F.A., Nurmatov A.A. Assessment and prediction of reproductive health of women of fertile age // Bulletin of the Academy of Medical Sciences of Tajikistan. 2019. T. 9. № 2 (30). C. 199-208.

92. Hamdamova M.T., Akhmatova D.F. Osteoporosis in young women of reproductive age, risk factors //Biology and Integrative Medicine 2021, 1(47), 146-159.

93. Hamdamova M.T. Age and individual variability of the shape and size of the uterus according to morphological and ultrasound studies// News of dermatovenerology and reproductive health. - 2020. - №1-2(88-80). - C. 49-52

94. Hikmatova S., Aslonova S.J. Modern ideas about polycystic ovary syndrome (PCOS) //Biology and Integrative Medicine 2017, 10(16), 4-22.

95. Khlyakina, O.V.; Gulin, A.V. Hygienic characterisation of the action of anthropogenic environmental factors on the state of health of the population of the Lipetsk region (in Russian) // Medico-social problems of modern Russia. Moscow, 2007. - C.92-97.

96. Khodjamuradova D.A., Nazalenko T.A. Endocrine forms of infertility in women in Tajikistan // Proceedings of the Academy of Sciences of the Republic of Tajikistan. Department of Biological and Medical Sciences, 2012, 1, 60-69.

97. Shodiev B.V., Mukhidova G.H. Microelementosis as a causal factor in the structure of reproductive losses// New Day in Medicine. - 2018. - №3(23). - C. 45-47.

98. Sholokhov L.F., Kolesnikova L.I., Dolgikh V.V. Restructuring of functional activity of the thyroid gland and therioid hormone metabolism in adolescent girls of different ethnic groups of Eastern Siberia as an important component of long-term adaptation to extreme climatic and geographical conditions of residence // Bulletin of the East Siberian Scientific Centre SB RAMS, 2013, 4, 77-80.

99. Shukurov F.A. Adaptation, stress and health Mat. 49th Scientific and Practical Conf. TSMU "Adaptation, Stress, Health", Dushanbe, 2001, pp.193-204.

100. Shukurov F.A. Interpersonal relations and vegetative status in the assessment of adaptation capabilities of students //

Health, demography, ecology of Finno-Ugric peoples. 2015. № 4. C. 65-68.

101. Shukurov F.A. Assessment and prediction of human adaptation capabilities to high altitude / In the collection: Ecological and physiological problems of adaptation. Proceedings of the XVII All-Russian symposium. 2017. C. 276-277.

102. Shukurov F.A. Assessment and prediction of individual forms of human adaptation to high altitude / Mat. I Interd.Conf. "Chronostructure and Chronology of Reproductive Function" and IX Interd.Conf. "Ecological and Physiological Mechanisms of Adaptation", Moscow, 2000, 233-235.

103. Shukurov F.A. Assessment and prediction of the effectiveness of human adaptation to high altitude / In Proceedings: Proceedings of the XXIII Congress of the I.P. Pavlov Physiological Society with international participation. 2017. C. 1503-1504.

104. Shukurov F.A. Physiological substantiation of criteria for assessment and prediction of individual adaptation of a person to high altitude. Dissertation abstract for a doctor of medical sciences. Moscow, 1995, 39 p.

105. Shukurov F.A., Arabzoda S.N. Characteristics of the forms of aggression and vegetative status in the assessment of adaptation capabilities of students //Vestnik of the Academy of Medical Sciences of Tajikistan. 2018. T. 8. № 1 (25), 111-117.

106. Shukurov F.A., Arabova Z.U. Vegetative status in the assessment of human adaptation to high-mountain hypoxia // Bulletin of the Academy of Medical Sciences of Tajikistan. 2018. T. 8. № 1 (25). C. 118-123.

107. Shukurov F.A., Arabova Z.U. Integral indicators of heart rate variability in the assessment of human adaptation to high altitude // Bulletin of the Academy of Medical Sciences of Tajikistan. 2019. T. 9. № 1 (29). C. 89-95.

108. Shukurov F.A., Arabova Z.U. Predicting the phase of stable adaptation and prenosological state in people with different length of residence in the high mountains // Proceedings of the National Academy of Sciences of the Kyrgyz Republic. 2019. - №4. - C. 83-87.

109. Shukurov F.A., Boboev A.A. The state of the autonomous nervous system in the assessment of health levels //

Applied Information Aspects of Medicine. 2015. T. 18. № 1. C. 212-220.

110. Shukurov F.A., Irgasheva D.Z. Body mass index and height-weight index in assessing the state of health of students //In the book: Agajanyanov Readings. Materials of II All-Russian scientific-practical conference. Dedicated to the 90th anniversary of the birth of Academician N.A. Aghajanyan. 2018. C. 304-306.

111. Shukurov F.A., Nidekker I.G. Dynamic structure of heart rhythm in the process of adaptation to high-altitude hypoxia //Cosmic Biology and Aerospace Medicine. 1981. № 3. C. 28.

112. Shukurov FA, Nidekker IG, Brodetskaya EE Individual features of the response of the cardiorespiratory system in humans during adaptation to high altitude // Human Physiology. 1991. T. 15. № 4. C. 105.

113. Shukurov F.A., Halimova F.T. Pre-nosological states of the body //Biology and Integrative Medicine 2019, 9(37), 68-80.

114. Shukurov F.A., Halimova F.T. Normal physiology Textbook for students of medical universities / Mauritius, 2020.

115. Shukurov F.A., Halimova F.T., Arabzoda S.N. Comparative characteristics of different forms of aggression with anxiety, correlation rhythmograms and functional state of the body // Bulletin of the Academy of Medical Sciences of Tajikistan. 2020. T. 10. № 2 (34). C. 196-201.

116. Shukurov FA, Halimova F.T., Arabova Z.U. Homeostasis indicators in short-term human adaptation to high altitude conditions and re-adaptation //Biology and Integrative Medicine 2020, 6(46), 5-22.

117. Shukurov F.A., Halimova F.T., Nurmatov A.A. Assessment and prediction of reproductive health of women of fertile age // Vestnik of the Academy of Medical Sciences of Tajikistan 2019, 9, 2(30), 199-208

118. Ermatov N.J., Abdulkhakov I.U. Socio-hygienic assessment of morbidity among different segments of the population on the materials of applications and in-depth medical examinations //Biology and Integrative Medicine 2021, 6(53), 472-488.

119. Yuldasheva D.Y., Usmonova A.O., Kayumova D.T. Comparative characteristics of the causes of recurrent dysfunctional uterine bleeding in premenopausal women //Biology and Integrative Medicine 2017, 2(8), 80-89.

120. Yakovenko N.V., Markov D.S. Environmental factors in the formation of health of the population of Ivanovo region (atmospheric air) // Modern Problems of Science and Education, 2013, 5, 461.

121. Adeel M., Song X., Wang Y.et al. Environmental impact of estrogens on human, animal and plant life: A critical review // . Int. 2017. Vol. 99, 107-119.

122. Agostinis C., Durigutto P., Sblattero D.et al. A non-complement-fixing antibody to β2 glycoprotein I as a novel therapy for antiphospholipid syndrome // Blood, 2014. - Vol. 123, N 22. - P. 3478-3487.

123. Akhmatova D.F., Khamdamova M.T. Analysis of the effectiveness of hormone therapy in patients with post-castration syndrome //Biology and Integrative Medicine 2021, 3(50), 27-33.

124. Akhmedov F.K. Peculiarities of cardiac hemodynamic in pregnant women with mild preeclampsia// Europen Science Review. - 2015. - №4-5. - C. 56 -58.

125. Akhmedov F.K. Role of study renal blood flow and concentration of uric acid in blood and urine in the diagnosis of preeclampsia //Biology and Integrative Medicine 2020, 2(42), 86-94.

126. Alijotas-Reig J., Llurba E., Gris J.M. Potentiating maternal immune tolerance in pregnancy: a new challenging role for regulatory T cells // Placenta, 2014. - Vol. 35, N 4. - P. 241-248.

127. Al-Saab R., Haddad S. Detection of thyroid autoimmunity markers in euthyroid women with polycystic ovary syndrome: a case-control study from Syria // Int. J. Endocrinol. Metab, 2014, Vol. 12, 3, 79-54.

128. Andreoli L., Chighizola C.B., Nalli C. et al. Clinical characterisation of antiphospholipid syndrome by detection of IgG antibodies against β_2 -glycoprotein i domain 1 and domain 4/5: ratio of anti-domain 1 to anti-domain 4/5 as a useful new biomarker for antiphospholipid syndrome // Arthritis Rheumatol. 2015. - Vol. 67, N 8. - P. 2196-2204.

129. Aquenor A., Bhatta-charya S. Infertility and miscarriage: common pathways in manifestation and management // Womens Health (Lond), 2015, Vol. 11, 4, 527-541.

130. Awoyemi T., Motta-Mejia C., Zhang W., Kouser L., White K., Kandzija N., Alhamlan F.S., Cribbs A.P., Tannetta D., Mazey E., Redman C., Kishore U., Vatish M. Syncytiotrophoblast Extracellular Vesicles From Late-Onset Preeclampsia Placentae

Suppress Pro-Inflammatory Immune Response in THP-1 Macrophages. //Front. Immunol. 2021, Jun 7, 12, 676056.

131. Barut M.U., Agacayak E., Bozkurt M. et al. There is a positive correlation between socioeconomic status and ovarian reserve in women of reproductive age // Med. Sci. Monit, 2016, Vol. 22, 4386-4392.

132. Bertolaccini M.L., Sanna G. Recent advances in understanding antiphospholipid syndrome // F1000 Res, 2016. - Vol. 5. - P. 2908-2923.

133. Bi M., Meng L., Bai L. Effects of Comprehensive Nursing Based on Orem's Self-Care Theory on Symptom Improvement and Pregnancy Outcome in Patients with Antiphospholipid Syndrome: A Retrospective Cohort Study. //Comput. Math. Methods Med. 2022, May 19, 2022:4133812.

134. Bliddal S., Boas M., Hilsted L. et al. Increase in thyroglobulin antibody and thyroid peroxidase antibody levels, but not preterm birth rate, in pregnant Danish women upon iodine fortification // Eur J Endocrinol, 2017, Vol. 176, 5, 603-612.

135. Busse M., Campe K.J., Redlich A., Oettel A., Hartig R., Costa S.D., Zenclussen A.C. Regulatory B Cells Are Decreased and Impaired in Their Function in Peripheral Maternal Blood in Preterm Birth. //Front. Immunol. 2020, Mar 20, 11, 386.

136. Busse M., Scharm M., Oettel A., Redlich A., Costa S.D., Zenclussen A.C. Enhanced S100B expression in T and B lymphocytes in spontaneous preterm birth and preeclampsia. //J. Perinat. Med. 2021, Nov 1, 50(2), 157-166.

137. Canaud G., Bienaimé F., Tabarin F. et al. Inhibition of the mTORC pathway in the antiphospholipid syndrome // N. Eng. Engl. J. Med. 2014, Vol. 371, 4, 303-312.

138. Carolan-Olah M., Frankowska D. High environmental temperature and preterm birth: a review of the evidence // Midwifery, 2014, Vol. 30, 1, 50-59.

139. Chen S., Liu Y., Sytwu H. Immunologic regulation in pregnancy: from mechanism to therapeutic strategy for immunomodulation // Clin. Develop. Immunol. 2012, Vol. 2012, 1-10.

140. Choudhury S.R., Knapp L.A. Human reproductive failure I immunological factors // Hum. Reprod. Update. 2001, Vol.7, 2, 113-134.

141. Christian L.M., Glaser R., Porter K., Iams J.D. Stress-induced inflammatory responses in women: effects of race and pregnancy // Psychosom. Med., 2013, Vol. 75, 7, 658-669.

142. Christiansen O.B.. Advances of intravenous immuneglobulin G in modulation of anti-fetal immunity in selected at-risk populations: science and therapeutics // Clin. Exp. Immunol, 2014, Vol. 178, 120-122.

143. Clark M.M., Chazara O., Sobel E.M. et al. Human birth weight and reproductive immunology: testing for interactions between maternal and offspring KIR and HLA-C genes //Hum Hered, 2017, Vol. 81, 4, 181-193.

144. Classen-Linke I., Mullen-Newen G. The cytokine-receptor GP 130 and its soluble form are under hormonal control in human endometrium and deciduas // Mol Hum Reprod, 2004. - Vol. 10. - P. 495-504.

145. Dadvand P., Wright J., Martinez D. et al. Inequality, green spaces, and pregnant women: roles of ethnicity and individual and neighbourhood socioeconomic status // Environ. Int, 2014, Vol. 71, 101-108.

146. De Carolis C., Perricone C., Perricone R. War and peace at the feto-placental front line: recurrent spontaneous abortion // Isr. Med. Assoc. J., 2014, Vol. 16, 10, 667-668.

147. Dewailly D., Andersen C.Y., Balen A. et al. The physiology and clinical utility of anti-Mullerian hormone in women // Hum. Reprod. Update, 2014, Vol. 20, 3, C. 370-385.

148. Donato J., Frazão R. Interactions between prolactin and kisspeptin to control reproduction // Arch. Endocrinol. Metab, 2016, Vol. 60, 6, 587-595.

149. Du V.X., Kelchtermans H., de Groot P.G. et al. From antibody to clinical phenotype, the black box of the antiphospholipid syndrome: pathogenic mechanisms of the antiphospholipid syndrome // Thromb. Res., 2013, Vol. 132, 3, 319-326.

150. Eastwood E.D., Kemp L., Jalaludin B. Explaining ecological clusters of maternal depression in South Western Sydney // BMC Pregnancy Childbirth, 2014, Vol. 14, 47.

151. Erlebacher A. Mechanisms of T cell tolerance towards the allogeneic fetus // Nat. Rev. Immunol, 2013, Vol. 13, 1, 23-33.

152. Findeklee S., Costa S.D., Tchaikovski S.N.. Thrombophilia and HELLP syndrome in pregnancy case report and overview of the literature // Z. Geburtshilfe Neonatol. Geburtshilfe Neonatol. 2015, Vol. 219, 1, 45-51.

153. Franchini M., Mannucci P.M. Impact on human health of climate changes // Eur. J. Intern. Med., 2015, Vol. 26, 1, 1-5.

154. Gailly-Fabre E., Kerlan V., Christin-Maitre S. [Pregnancy-associated hormones and fetal-maternal relations] // Ann. Endocrinol. (Paris), 2015, Vol. 76, 6, Suppl 1, 39-50.

155. Ghaebi M., Nouri M., Ghasemzadeh A. et al. Immune regulatory network in successful pregnancy and reproductive failures // Biomed. Pharmacother. 2017, Vol. 88, 61-73.

156. Gleicher N., Weghofer A., Barad D.H.. Cutting edge assessment of the impact of autoimmunity on female reproductive success // J. Autoimmun. Autoimmun. 2012, Vol. 38, 74-80.

157. Gonzales G.F., Zevallos A., Gonzales-Castañeda C. et al. Environmental pollution, climate variability and climate change: a review of health impacts on the Peruvian population // Rev. Peru Med. Exp. Salud. Publica, 2014, Vol. 31, 3, 547-556.

158. Green D. Pathophysiology of Antiphospholipid Syndrome. //Thromb. Haemost. 2021, Nov 18.

159. Grimstad F., Krieg S. Immunogenetic contributions to recurrent pregnancy loss // J. Assist. Reprod. Genet. 2016, Vol. 33, 7, 833-847.

160. Harris R., Cormack D., Stanley J., Rameka R. Investigating the relationship between ethnic consciousness, racial discrimination and self-rated health in New Zealand // PLoS One, 2015, Vol. 10, N 2. - P. 317-343.

161. He Y., Pan A., Yang Y. et al. Prevalence of underweight, overweight, and obesity among reproductive-age women and adolescent girls in Rural China // Am. J. Public. Health, 2016, Vol. 106, 12, 2103-2110.

162. Heyn H., Moran S., Hernando-Herraez I. et al. DNA methylation contributes to natural human variation // Genome Res. 2013, Vol. 23, 9, 1363-1372.

163. Hsiang J., Selvaratnam S., Taylor S. et al. Increasing primary antibiotic resistance and ethnic differences in eradication rates of Helicobacter pylori infection in New Zealand a new look at an old enemy // N.Z. Med. J., 2013, Vol. 126, 1384, 64-76.

164. Ivarsson M.A., Stiglund N., Marquardt N. et al. Composition and dynamics of the uterine NK cell KIR repertoire in menstrual blood // Mucosal. Immunol, 2017. Vol. 10, 2, 322-331.

165. Jiang T.T., Chaturvedi V., Ertelt J.M. et al. Regulatory T cells: new keys for further unlocking the enigma of fetal tolerance

and pregnancy complications // J. Immunol. Immunol. 2014. - Vol. 192, N 11. - P. 4949-4956.

166. Khamdamov I.B. A differentiated approach to the choice of diagnostics and prevention of complications of prosthetic plasty in women of fertile age //Biology and Integrative Medicine 2022, 1(54), 5-14.

167. Khamdamova M.T. Age echographic characteristics of the uterus and ovaries in women of the first and second period of middle age //Biology and Intcgrative Medicine 2020, 2(42), 75-85.

168. Khamdamova M.T. Echographic features of the range of variability in the size of the uterus and ovaries in women of menopausal age using oral and injectable forms of contraception/American Journal of Medicine and Medical Sciences. - 2020. - N10 (8). - P. 580- 583.

169. Khamdamova M.T., Teshaev Sh.J., Haribova E.A., Ikhtiyarova G.A. Features of ultrasound diagnostics of inflammatory processes of the uterus and appendages when using intrauterine contraceptives in women living in the Bukhara region // Biology and Integrative Medicine 2020, 5(45), 76-94.

170. Khatamova M.T., Burkhanova M.E., Fayzulloeva N.Sh. Aspects of delivery during the prenatal discharge of amniotic fluid //Biology and Integrative Medicine 2021, 1(47), 110-120.

171. Kholova N.F., Khamdamova M.T.. Diagnosis of reproductive health disorders in girls of early reproductive age //Biology and Integrative Medicine 2021, 5(52), 34-41.

172. Kiely M., A.A.El-Mohandes, M.G.Gantz et al. Understanding the association of biomedical, psychosocial and behavioural risks with adverse pregnancy outcomes among African-Americans in Washington, DC // Matern. Child. Health J. 2011, Vol. 15, Suppl 1, 85-95.

173. Kim K., Bloom M.S., Browne R.W. et al. Associations between follicular fluid high density lipoprotein particle components and embryo quality among in vitro fertilisation patients // J. Assist. Assist. Reprod. Genet. 2017, Vol. 34, 1, 1-10.

174. Kjellstrom T. Impact of climate conditions on occupational health and related economic losses: A new feature of global and urban health in the context of climate change // Asia Pac. J. Public. Health. 2016. - Vol. 28, 2 Suppl., 28-37.

175. Knight J.S., Kanthi Y. Mechanisms of immunothrombosis and vasculopathy in antiphospholipid syndrome. //Semin. Immunopathol. 2022, May, 44(3), 347-362.

176. Kövér Á., Lampé R., Szabó K., Tarr T., Papp G. A Comprehensive Investigation into the Distribution of Circulating B Cell Subsets in the Third Trimester of Pregnancy. //J. Clin. Med. 2022, May 26, 11(11), 3006.

177. Koyuncu T., Metintas S., Ayhan E. et al. Evaluation of reproductive health criteria in seasonal agricultural workers: a sample from Eskisehir, Turkey // Rural. Remote Health, 2016, Vol. 16, 4, 3489.

178. Kust A.V., Sotnikova N.Y., Malyshkina A.I., Voronin D.N.. Role of CD20 + IL-10 + B-lymphocytes in immunoregulatory processes in women with reccurent miscarriage. //Klin. Lab. Diagn. 2021, Aug 13, 66(8), 485-488.

179. Kwak-Kim J., Skariah A., Wu L. et al. Humoral and cellular autoimmunity in women with recurrent pregnancy losses and repeated implantation failures: A possible role of vitamin D// Autoimmun. Rev, 2016, Vol. 15, 10, 943-947.

180. La Rocca C., Carbone F., Longobardi S., Matarese G. The immunology of pregnancy: regulatory T cells control maternal immune tolerance towards the fetus // Immunol. Lett, 2014, Vol. 162, 1, Pt A., 41-48.

181. Lacorcia M., Bhattacharjee S., Laubhahn K., Alhamdan F., Ram M., Muschaweckh A., Potaczek D.P., Kosinska A., Garn H., Protzer U., Renz H., Prazeres da Costa C. Fetomaternal immune cross talk modifies T-cell priming through sustained changes to DC function. //J. Allergy Clin. Immunol. 2021, Sep., 148(3), 843-857.

182. Lassi Z.S., Middleton P.F., Bhutta Z.A., Crowther C. Strategies for improving health care see-king for maternal and newborn illnesses in low- and middle-income countries: a systematic review and meta-analysis // Glob. Health. Action. 2016, Vol. 9, 1, 31408.

183. Lawson A.K., Marsh E.E.. Hearing the silenced voices of under-served women: The role of qualitative research in gynecologic and reproductive care // Obstet. Gynecol. Clin. North Am, 2017, Vol. 44, 1, 109-120.

184. Lee S.K., Kim C.J., Kim D.J., Kang J.H.. Immune cells in the female reproductive tract // Immune Netw, 2015,Vol. 15, 1, 16-26.

185. Lin X., Liang Q., Lin L. et al. Identification of antimyosin antibodies in the serums of patients with antiphospholipid syndrome// Thromb. Res, 2015, Vol.135, 5, 867-872.

186. Liu J.J., Davidson E., Bhopal R., White M., Johnson M., Netto G., Sheikh A.. Adapting health promotion interventions for ethnic minority groups: a qualitative study// Health Promot. Int. 2016, Vol. 31, 2, 325-334.

187. Liu N., Chen J., He Y., Jia H., Jiang D., Li S., Yang Y., Dai Z., Wu Z., Wu G. Effects of maternal L-proline supplementation on inflammatory cytokines at the placenta and fetus interface of mice. //Amino Acids. 2020, Apr., 52(4), 587-596.

188. Londra L.C., Tobler K.J, Omurtag K.R., Donohue M.B.. Spanish language content on reproductive endocrinology and infertility practice websites // Fertil. Steril. 2014, Vol. 102, 5, 1371-1376.

189. Maaki S.M., Nick S., Macklon J., Coboi J. Embryonic implantation: cytokines, adhesion molecules and immune cells in establishing an implantation environment // J. Leukocytes. Leukoc. Biol. 2009, Vol. 85, 1, 4-19.

190. Magatti M., Masserdotti A., Cargnoni A., Papait A., Stefani F.R., Silini A.R., Parolini O. The Role of B Cells in PE Pathophysiology: A Potential Target for Perinatal Cell-Based Therapy //Int. J. Mol. Sci. 2021, Mar 26, 22(7), 3405. doi: 10.3390/ijms22073405.

191. Manukyan G., Martirosyan A., Slavik L., Ulehlova J., Dihel M., Papajik T., Kriegova E. 17β-Estradiol Promotes Proinflammatory and Procoagulatory Phenotype of Innate Immune Cells in the Presence of Antiphospholipid Antibodies. //Biomedicines. 2020, Jun 15, 8(6), 162.

192. Mavlyanova N.N., Ikhtiyarova G.I., Tosheva I.I., Aslonova M.Zh., Narzullaeva N.S. The State of the Cytokine Status in Pregnant Women with Fetal Growth Retardation// Journal of Medical - Clinical Research & Reviews. ISSN 2639 - 944X. - 2020, №4(6), 18-22.

193. Monteiro C., Kasahara T., Sacramento P.M., Dias A., Leite S., Silva V.G., Gupta S., Agrawal A., Bento C.A.M. Human pregnancy levels of estrogen and progesterone contribute to humoral immunity by activating T_{FH} /B cell axis. //Eur. J. Immunol. 2021, Jan., 51(1), 167-179.

194. Muller A.F., Berghout A. Consequences of autoimmune thyroiditis before, during and after pregnancy // Minerva Endocrinol, 2003, Vol. 28, 3,247-254.

195. Muzzio D., Zenclussen A.C., Jensen F. The role of B cells in pregnancy: the good and the bad // Am. J. Reprod. Immunol. 2013, Vol. 69, 4, 408-412.

196. Nalli C., Tincani A. Pregnancy in antiphospholipid syndrome: can we improve patient management? // Isr. Med. Assoc. J. 2014, Vol. 16, 10, 614-615.

197. Palmeira P.. Quinello C., Silveira-Lessa A.L. et al. IgG placental transfer in healthy and pathological pregnancies // Clin. Dev. Immunol. 2012, Vol. 2012, 1-13.

198. Panova I.A., Kudryashova A.V., Panashchatenko A.S., Rokotyanskaya E.A., Malyshkina A.I., Parejshvili V.V., Harlamova N.V. Character of β-lymphocytes differentiation in women with hypertensive disorders during pregnancy. //Klin. Lab. Diagn. 2021, Aug 13, 66(8), 489-495.

199. Paterson J., Berry P., Ebi K., Varangu L. Health care facilities resilient to climate change impacts // Int. J. Environ. Res. Publ. Health, 2014, Vol. 1, 12, 113-116.

200. Piccinni M.P., Lombardelli L., Logiodice F. et al. How pregnancy can affect autoimmune diseases progression? // Clin. Mol. Allergy, 2016, Vol. 14, 11-22.

201. Ponce A., Rodríguez-Pintó I., Basauli J.M., Espinosa G., Erkan D., Shoenfeld Y., Cervera R; On Behalf of the CAPS Registry Project Group/European Forum on Antiphospholipid Antibodies. The clinical significance of low complement levels in patients with catastrophic antiphospholipid syndrome: A descriptive analysis of 73 patients from the "Catastrophic antiphospholipid syndrome registry". //Lupus. 2022, Jun 10, 9612033221107583.

202. Posch F., Gebhart J., Rand J.H. et al. Cardiovascular risk factors are major determinants of thrombotic risk in patients with the lupus anti-coagulant // BMC Med. 2017, Vol. 15, 54-66.

203. Rabiev S.N., Teshaev Sh.J., Khamdamova M.T., Haribova E.A. Features of anthropometric indicators of fetal development in women of different somatotypes //Biology and Integrative Medicine 2021, 3(50), 34-46.

204. Rebello K., Silva J., Brito R.C.S. Fundamental factors in marital satisfaction: An assessment of Brazilian couples // Psychology, 2014, Vol. 5, 7, 777-784.

205. Rocheleau C.M., Bertke S.J., Lawson C.C. et all. Factors associated with employment status before and during pregnancy: Implications for studies of pregnancy outcomes // Am. J. Ind. Med. 2017, Vol. 60, 4, 329-341.

206. Rosa Dos Santos A.P., de Oliveira Vaz C., Hounkpe B.W., Jacintho B.C., Oliveira J.D., Tripiquia Vechiatto Mesquita G.L., Pereira Dos Santos I., Annichino-Bizzacchi J., Appenzeller S., de Moraes Mazetto Fonseca B., Orsi F.A. Association between interferon-I producing plasmacytoid dendritic cells and thrombotic antiphospholipid syndrome. //Lupus. 2022, May 25, 9612033221101731.

207. Rosenblum M.D., Way S.S., Abbas A.K.. Regulatory T cell memory // Nat. Rev. Immunol. 2016, Vol. 16, 2, 90-101.

208. Rylander C., Odland J.O., Sandanger T.M. Climate change and the potential effects on maternal and pregnancy outcomes: an assessment of the most vulnerable--the mother, fetus, and newborn child // Glob. Health. Action. 2013, Vol. 6, 195-198.

209. Sarfaty M., Mitchell M., Bloodhart B., Maibach E.W.. A survey of African American physicians on the health effects of climate change // Int. J. Environ. Res. Publ. Health, 2014, Vol. 11, 12, 173-185.

210. Schander J.A., Marvaldi C., Correa F., Wolfson M.L., Cella M., Aisemberg J., Jensen F., Franchi A.M. Maternal environmental enrichment modulates the immune response against an inflammatory challenge during gestation and protects the offspring. //J. Reprod. Immunol. 2021, Apr., 144, 103273.

211. Scholz P., Auler M., Brachvogel B. et al. Detection of multiple annexin autoantibodies in a patient with recurrent miscarriages, fulminant stroke and seronegative antiphospholipid syndrome // Biochem. Med. (Zagreb), 2016. Vol. 26, 2, 272-278.

212. Sciascia S., Sanna G., Murru V. et al. Anti-prothrombin (aPT) and antiphosphatidyl-serine/prothrombin (aPS/PT) antibodies and the risk of thrombosis in the antiphospholipid syndrome. A systematic review // Thromb. Haemost. 2014, Vol. 111, 2, 354-364.

213. Skjærvø G.R., Fossøy F., Røskaft E.Solar activity at birth predicted infant survival and women's fertility in historical Norway // . Biol. Sci, 2015, Vol. 282, 1801, 2014-2032.

214. Slawek A., Lorek D., Kedzierska A.E., Chelmonska-Soyta A. Regulatory B cells with IL-35 and IL-10 expression in a

normal and abortion-prone murine pregnancy model. //Am. J. Reprod. Immunol. 2020, Mar., 83(3), e13217.

215. Sletner L., Nakstad B., Yajnik C.S. et al. Ethnic differences in neonatal body composition in a multi-ethnic population and the impact of parental factors: a population-based cohort study // PLoS One, 2013, Vol. 8, 8, 730-758.

216. Sonecha S., Noble A.J., Morgan M., Ridsdale L. Perceptions and experiences of epilepsy among patients from black ethnic groups in South London // Prim. Health Care Res. Dev. 2014, Vol. 15, 1-11.

217. Southcombe J.H., Redman C.W., Sargent I.L., Granne I. IL-1 family cytokines and their regulatory proteins in normal pregnancy and pre-eclampsia/ J.H.Southcombe, // Clin. Exp. Immunol. 2015, Vol. 181, 3, 480-490.

218. Staun-Ram E., Shalev E. Human trophoblast function during the implantation process // Reprod Biol Endocrinol, 2005, Vol. 3, 56-67.

219. Stouffs K., Seneca S., Lissens W. Genetic causes of male infertility // Ann. Endocrinol. (Paris), 2014, Vol. 75, 2, 109-111.

220. Thayaparan A.S. Lowe S.A.. Cutaneous pseudovasculitis, anti-phospholipid syndrome and obstetric misadventure // Lupus, 2015, Vol. 24, 10, 1107-1110.

221. Tincani A., Dall'Ara F., Lazzaroni M.G. Pregnancy in patients with autoimmune disease: A reality in 2016 // Autoimmun. Rev. 2016, Vol. 15, 10, 975-977.

222. Ulrich V. Gelber S.E., Vukelic M. et al. ApoE Receptor 2 Mediation of Trophoblast Dysfunction and Pregnancy Complications Induced by Antiphospholipid Antibodies in Mice // Arthritis Rheumatol. 2016. - Vol. 68, N 3. - P. 730-739.

223. Urbanus R.T., Pennings M.T., Derksen R.H. et al. Platelet activation by dimeric beta2-glycoprotein I requires signalling via both glycoprotein Ibalpha and apolipoprotein E receptor 2' // J. Thromb. Thromb. Haemost. 2008, Vol. 6, 8, 1405-1412.

224. Valeff N., Muzzio D.O., Matzner F., Dibo M., Golchert J., Homuth G., Abba M.C., Zygmunt M., Jensen F. B cells acquire a unique and differential transcriptomic profile during pregnancy. //Genomics. 2021, Jul., 113(4), 2614-2622.

225. Valeff N.J., Ventimiglia M.S., Dibo M., Markert U.R., Jensen F. Splenic B1 B Cells Acquire a Proliferative and

Anti-Inflammatory Profile During Pregnancy in Mice. //Front. Immunol. 2022, Apr 28, 13:873493.

226. Wakeel F., Witt W.P., Wisk L.E. et al. Racial and ethnic disparities in personal capital during pregnancy: findings from the 2007 Los Angeles mommy and baby (LAMB) study // Matter. Child. health J. 2014, Vol. 18(1), 209-222.

227. Wang W.J., Liu F.J., Xin-Liu et al. Adoptive transfer of pregnancy-induced CD4+CD25+ regulatory T cells reverses the increase in abortion rate caused by interleukin 17 in the CBA/JxBALB/c mouse model // Hum. Reprod. 2014, Vol. 29, 5, 946-952.

228. Warembourg C., Debost-Legrand A., Bonvallot N. et al. Exposure of pregnant women to persistent organic pollutants and cord sex hormone levels // Hum. Reprod. 2016, Vol. 31, 1, 190-198.

229. Yan H., Li B., Su R., Gao C., Li X., Wang C.. Preliminary Study on the Imbalance Between Th17 and Regulatory T Cells in Antiphospholipid Syndrome. //Front. Immunol. 2022, May 6, 13:873644.

230. Zhai X., Yang S., Cui L. Anticardiolipin IgA as a Potential Risk Factor for Pregnancy Morbidity in Patients with Antiphospholipid Syndrome. //Lab. Med. 2022, May 29, lmac028.

231. Zhu R., Cheng C.Y., Yang Y., Denas G., Pengo V. Prevalence of aPhosphatidylserine/prothrombin antibodies and association with antiphospholipid antibody profiles in patients with antiphospholipid syndrome: A systematic review and meta-analysis. //Thromb. Res. 2022, Jun., 214, 106-114.

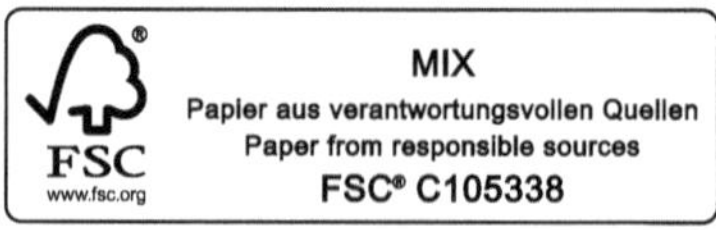

Printed by Books on Demand GmbH, Norderstedt / Germany